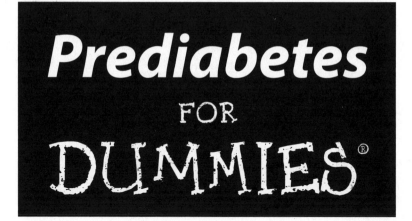

Prediabetes
FOR
DUMMIES®

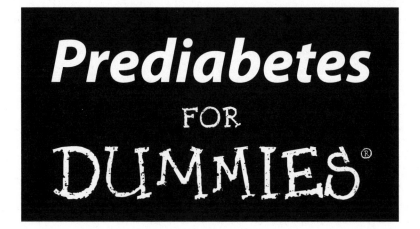

Prediabetes FOR DUMMIES®

by Alan L. Rubin, MD

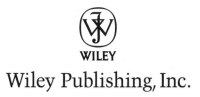

WILEY

Wiley Publishing, Inc.

Prediabetes For Dummies®

Published by
Wiley Publishing, Inc.
111 River St.
Hoboken, NJ 07030-5774
www.wiley.com

WILEY

About the Author

Alan L. Rubin, M.D., is one of the nation's foremost experts on diabetes. He is a professional member of the American Diabetes Association and the Endocrine Society and has been in private practice specializing in diabetes and thyroid disease for over 30 years. Dr. Rubin was Assistant Clinical Professor of Medicine at University of California Medical Center in San Francisco for 20 years. He has spoken about diabetes to professional medical audiences and non-medical audiences around the world. He has been a consultant to many pharmaceutical companies and companies that make diabetes products.

Dr. Rubin was one of the first specialists in his field to recognize the significance of patient self-testing of blood glucose, the major advance in diabetes care since the advent of insulin. As a result, he has been on numerous radio and television programs, talking about the cause, the prevention, and the treatment of diabetes and its complications.

Since publishing *Diabetes For Dummies,* Dr. Rubin has had four other bestselling *For Dummies* books — *Diabetes Cookbook For Dummies, Thyroid For Dummies, High Blood Pressure For Dummies,* and *Type 1 Diabetes For Dummies* — all published by Wiley Publishing. These four books cover the medical problems of 100 million Americans.

Dedication

This book is dedicated to my new granddaughter, Rachel Natania Ross, who was born almost exactly when the book was completed. It is my fervent hope that she will never need the information in it, but if so, that it contains all she needs to know to live a long, healthy, active life.

Author's Acknowledgments

For this first edition, acquisitions editor Michael Lewis deserves major thanks. I have had the pleasure of working with him for several years. He is supportive, encouraging, and fun and I look forward to a long association with him. I am also blessed with another great project editor, Joan Friedman, who not only made sure that everything was readable and understandable, but offered excellent suggestions to improve the information. My thanks also to Dr. Dawn Ayers for reviewing the book.

Publisher's Acknowledgments

We're proud of this book; please send us your comments at http://dummies.custhelp.com. For other comments, please contact our Customer Care Department within the U.S. at 877-762-2974, outside the U.S. at 317-572-3993, or fax 317-572-4002.

Some of the people who helped bring this book to market include the following:

Acquisitions, Editorial, and Media Development

Project Editor: Joan Friedman

Acquisitions Editor: Michael Lewis

Assistant Editor: Erin Calligan Mooney

Editorial Program Coordinator: Joe Niesen

Technical Editor: Dawn M. Ayers, MD

Senior Editorial Manager: Jennifer Ehrlich

Editorial Supervisor: Carmen Krikorian

Editorial Assistants: David Lutton, Jennette ElNaggar

Art Coordinator: Alicia B. South

Cover Photos: © iStock

Cartoons: Rich Tennant (www.the5thwave.com)

Illustrations: Kathryn Born, M.A.

Composition Services

Project Coordinator: Patrick Redmond

Layout and Graphics: Melissa K. Jester, Christine Williams

Proofreaders: Jessica Kramer, Linda Seifert

Indexer: Slivoskey Indexing Services

Publishing and Editorial for Consumer Dummies

> **Diane Graves Steele,** Vice President and Publisher, Consumer Dummies

> **Kristin Ferguson-Wagstaffe,** Product Development Director, Consumer Dummies

> **Ensley Eikenburg,** Associate Publisher, Travel

> **Kelly Regan,** Editorial Director, Travel

Publishing for Technology Dummies

> **Andy Cummings,** Vice President and Publisher, Dummies Technology/General User

Composition Services

> **Debbie Stailey,** Director of Composition Services

Contents at a Glance

Table of Contents

Introduction

· ·

We're going to have some fun together. "What," you say, "is funny about a discussion of a problem like prediabetes?" On the surface, maybe nothing. But a spoonful of humor makes the medicine go down. If you ask women what they want in a man, a majority will say "a sense of humor" (among other things). I believe that's what you want in a book as well. I believe you will find what I have to tell you much more palatable if I add a dash of fun. If it's too dry, you won't be able to swallow it. So prepare to smile.

Why Do We Need This Book?

The simple answer is that my wife wants to redo the bathroom. But, as you can imagine, the answer is much more complex. The prefix *pre* means "before," as in *prefix*, "before the word." *Prediabetes* is that time when you aren't quite normal but you don't quite have diabetes. I define it clearly in Chapter 1. Prediabetes is not usually associated with all the bad complications of diabetes, which I discuss in Chapters 12, 13, and 14, but it may be associated with some heart problems, which I discuss in Chapter 13.

And prediabetes is not only the stage before diabetes. It may also be the stage before high blood pressure (*prehypertension*) and the stage before high cholesterol (*precholesterol*: Oh, sorry, I got carried away — there is no such term). All the abnormalities that lead to prediabetes (that can go on to diabetes) are also to blame for the development of prehypertension (that can go on to high blood pressure) and mildly elevated cholesterol (that can go on to hypercholesterolemia).

So if I help you to reverse prediabetes, I am also helping you to reverse the other two conditions. You are basically getting three books for the price of one. What a deal!

And you *can* reverse prediabetes. If there is one thing that I want to make clear, you are not doomed to develop diabetes just because you have prediabetes. You can return to your normal state of perfection. But you have to read what I have written, and you have to follow my recommendations. If you reverse prediabetes, you will probably reverse prehypertension and mildly elevated cholesterol as well. Chapters 15 through 20 provide everything you need to know to do this.

About This Book

This book is an excellent resource for what you need to know about prediabetes — and a lot about diabetes as well. (Everything you need to know about diabetes can be found in an excellent book called *Diabetes For Dummies,* written by an author well-known to me and published by Wiley.)

You don't have to read this book from start to finish (but it wouldn't hurt). You can pick up the book and start reading anywhere you want. If you want to know what prediabetes is, start with Chapter 1. If you want to know what factors lead to prediabetes, Part II provides the answers. Getting a diagnosis is taken up in Part III, while the potential complications should you develop diabetes are discussed in Part IV. Part V tells you how to avoid or reverse prediabetes.

So if you are some kind of genius and already know what prediabetes is, how to diagnose it, and that you have it, go ahead and skip to Part V. But be forewarned! I will ask you to do things that may be a lot harder than tenth-grade math. Unlike tenth-grade math, however, what I ask you to do can save and prolong your life. Just avoid getting hit by a car.

Conventions Used in This Book

The sugar in your blood is called *glucose,* and too-high glucose leads to many of the complications of diabetes. But the white sugar you eat is not glucose; it's sucrose. And many other sugars exist, like fructose, maltose, and galactose. So I don't use just the word *sugar* in this book; I call the particular sugar by its proper name.

When I mention a level of blood sugar (oops, glucose), it will be shown in units called *milligrams per deciliter* (mg/dl). I don't mean to confuse you, but the rest of the world uses the International System of units called, in this case, *millimoles per liter* (mmol/L). You can convert mg/dl to mmol/L as you cross the border of the United States into Canada simply by dividing the mg/dl by 18. For example, a blood glucose of 100 mg/dl is 5.5 mmol/L.

Two major types of diabetes exist: *type 1* diabetes mellitus and *type 2* diabetes mellitus. I refer to them as *type 1* and *type 2* diabetes in this book.

I discuss calories frequently in this book because how many of them you eat affects your weight, which in turn affects your susceptibility to prediabetes and diabetes. When I talk about a specific number of calories that you consume, I use the proper term, which is *kilocalorie. A calorie* is actually a much smaller unit of energy than a kilocalorie. Food manufacturers always use the abbreviated *calorie,* which is confusing and not technically correct.

Finally, in Chapter 16, I include a handful of recipes to try. If you're a vegetarian, look for the tomato next to the recipe name that indicates the recipe does not contain meat or fish.

What You Don't Have to Read

You don't have to read anything in this book if you don't want to, but that would be a waste of my time and your money. Instead, if you really don't like complicated scientific explanations, skip the material in the sidebars that are shaded in grey. You will still understand everything else, but you may not be able to answer a trivia question someday. The sidebars are there for the people who demand to know why.

Foolish Assumptions

I assume that your mind is a blank when it comes to prediabetes and diabetes. Therefore, you won't suddenly come up against a term that you have never seen before without finding an immediate definition of that term. On the other hand, if you already know something about the subject, you can expect to find much greater detail. Throughout the book, the most important points are clearly marked using tools such as icons (which I explain in a moment).

How This Book Is Organized

This book has six parts, and you don't have to start at Part I. Each part is self-contained. In fact, each chapter is self-contained, so if you see a chapter title that really excites you like "The Testing Spectrum: Having the Essential Tests and Interpreting Results," feel free to jump right in there. Here is a brief discussion of what you can find in each part of this book.

Part 1: Confronting the Prediabetes Epidemic

This introductory part gives you a foundation of understanding as to what prediabetes is all about. I start with a discussion of how prediabetes originates. From there, I move on to talk about when you should suspect that you have developed prediabetes. What are the elements of your family history, your personal history, and your current lifestyle that suggest this diagnosis?

Moving right along, I trace the factors that convert prediabetes to diabetes. Then I offer a general discussion about stopping this conversion before it happens.

Part II: Food and Other Factors: Battling an Unhealthy Lifestyle

What you learn in these chapters should make it clear to you that prediabetes, as well as type 2 diabetes, is promoted by an unhealthy lifestyle, which means both conditions can be reversed by adopting a healthy lifestyle.

The first element of your lifestyle to consider is the food you eat. Some foods are good for you, and others aren't. You constantly make choices, and I want to help you make the right ones. From your own kitchen to the homes of your friends to the restaurants you frequent, you need to be aware of what to choose.

Next you want to deal with your weight. I am not interested in turning you into a fashion model, just getting your weight to the level where it does not hurt your health. Of course, should you decide to turn into a fashion model, I wouldn't mind a signed photograph.

The next aspect of your lifestyle that we must deal with is your exercise program. What exercise program, you say? If you don't exercise, that has got to change. You want to feel all those good chemicals that come from your brain when you exercise. It's a natural, inexpensive, and very healthful high.

Finally, you want to learn how to deal with stress so it doesn't damage your health, and you want to eliminate bad habits such as any interaction with tobacco of any kind, as well as excessive drinking. I help you to do those things to the best of my ability, but you have to carry them out (so they don't carry you out).

Part III: Getting a Diagnosis

First I want to help you recognize what is going wrong. Diabetes, and even more so prediabetes, is like a stealth bomber. You may not see it coming before a lot of damage is done.

Many tests can be valuable both to make the diagnosis of prediabetes and to see how far along you are. I explain these tests in detail and tell you when to get them and how to interpret them. You may be able to teach your doctor a thing or two before you finish this part.

Special issues apply to children and the elderly when it comes to diagnosing prediabetes. The final chapter in this part discusses these issues. We are witnessing an epidemic of type 2 diabetes in children, which means there is an even greater epidemic of prediabetes in children. Is that excess weight just baby fat that will disappear when your child has a growth spurt? Or is it necessary to do something right now to help your child get healthy? You find out here.

Part IV: The Dangers of Moving toward Diabetes

Diabetes, untreated, is not a benign condition. People with diabetes are the largest component of blind people and people with kidney failure in the United States. This part clarifies the complications, both major and minor, that are associated with uncontrolled diabetes.

First there are the short-term complications that can come and go in a few days or even hours, such as low blood glucose (*hypoglycemia*) and very high blood glucose (*hyperglycemia*). These conditions have a very definite effect on your quality of life and need to be prevented.

Next are the long-term complications that take ten or more years of diabetes to develop but can be devastating. Blindness, kidney failure, nerve disease, and heart disease are the things to fear in this regard. But you are never going to have any of these complications because you are going to reverse your prediabetes so it never gets to diabetes!

A special category of long-term complications are sexual complications and the complications of pregnancy. These situations warrant their own chapter. (It's not X-rated, so feel free to read it even when the kids are around.)

Part V: Avoiding or Reversing Prediabetes

Up to now you have been learning. Now you will be doing, with my help. First, in Chapter 15, we go to the supermarket together and make good choices. Then we cook together and enjoy the healthful and delicious food we make. In Chapter 16, I provide you with a bunch of recipes that you can enjoy — recipes that feature inexpensive ingredients so anyone can make them.

Next I take up exercise. You may find some surprises in Chapter 17, but you have to read it to find them out. I am not giving you any clues here.

Can medications help to reverse prediabetes? You find out in Chapter 18, and you also learn whether any vitamins or supplements may make a difference.

Surgery for weight loss may seem like a drastic solution, but it may not be as drastic as you think. When all else fails, this option is a reasonable and almost guaranteed answer. You find out how surgery may help, its pros and cons, and what to expect if you have weight loss surgery in Chapter 19.

To put all your new knowledge together, I provide Chapter 20, which features a complete plan for a three-month health makeover. Sometimes you need structure in order to succeed. This chapter tells you what to eat, what exercise to do, and everything else you need to know.

Part VI: The Part of Tens

No book *For Dummies* is complete without this part. You can read ten myths about prediabetes, ten staples to keep in your kitchen, and ten things to teach your child with prediabetes.

Icons Used in This Book

The icons alert you to information you must know, information you should know, and information you may find interesting but can live without.

I use this icon when I relate a story from my personal experience or from the experience of one of my patients.

This icon points out when you should see your doctor (for example, if your blood glucose level is too high or you need a particular test done).

When you see this icon, it means the information is essential and you should be aware of it.

This icon marks important information that can save you time and energy.

Part I

Confronting the Prediabetes Epidemic

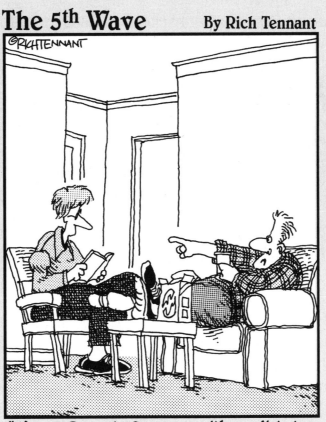

The 5th Wave   By Rich Tennant

"C'mon, Darryl! Someone with prediabetes shouldn't be lying around all day. Whereas someone with no life, like myself, has a very good reason."

In this part . . .

Prediabetes is a relatively new concept. In this part I explain its meaning and who is affected. I tell you how to recognize that you or a loved one may have prediabetes. I discuss the transition from prediabetes to diabetes. And I open the discussion of how to stop prediabetes from becoming diabetes and how to return your metabolism to its normal state.

Chapter 1

The Origins and Dangers of Prediabetes

About 60 million people in the United States have prediabetes. That means if you are in a room with three other adult U.S. citizens, one of you will probably have prediabetes, and chances are that person won't know it. The purpose of this book is to radically change that situation. Anyone who reads this book will know whether he or she has prediabetes. Anyone who follows the recommendations in this book will *not* proceed to diabetes and will probably return to normal health.

This book will not make you younger, but it will help you continue to get older.

Diagnosing prediabetes is crucial because prediabetes is the critical step before developing diabetes. As you find out in this book, diabetes is associated with complications that may cause considerable physical and mental discomfort at best and be life-threatening at worst. So you don't want to go there.

Even if you go on to develop diabetes, all is not lost. You can use the suggestions found here to avoid further complications. You can't get rid of the diagnosis, but you can get rid of the problems.

In this chapter, you discover how to differentiate among three physical states: normal health, prediabetes, and diabetes. I explain that prediabetes is a recent phenomenon, which parallels the epidemic of obesity and lack of exercise in the United States and around the world.

Next, you discover who is affected by prediabetes and which groups of people are at the highest risk. I also touch on special considerations for children and the elderly at risk for prediabetes.

Finally, I focus on the costs of prediabetes, which are not only monetary. I explain that even though prediabetes is often considered a benign condition and not a disease, changes occur in the body of a person with prediabetes that may not be benign after all.

Distinguishing Prediabetes from Diabetes

Jane Johnson is a 48-year-old woman. She is postmenopausal and has gained about 15 pounds since her twenties, when her weight was normal. She complains of some fatigue. She goes to Dr. Sugarfeld, who discovers that Jane has family members with diabetes. Jane mentions that she used to be physically active but doesn't have the time to do much exercise these days. A physical examination reveals only that Jane is overweight and has mild high blood pressure, so Dr. Sugarfeld sends her for blood tests. One of the blood tests the doctor orders is called a *fasting blood glucose,* and it discovers the level of sugar in someone's blood in the morning after that person has fasted through the night.

When Jane returns a week later, Dr. Sugarfeld informs her that her fasting blood glucose was 114 mg/dl (6.3 mmol/L). (In the Introduction to this book, I explain what *mg/dl* and *mmol/L* stand for, in case you're interested.) The doctor asks Jane to have one more fasting blood glucose test. This value is 108 mg/dl (6 mmol/L). Dr Sugarfeld informs Jane that she has prediabetes.

Going from normal to prediabetes

This anecdote describes one of the most common ways that prediabetes is discovered. Another common occurrence is simply the discovery that the *blood glucose* — the amount of sugar in the blood — is higher than it should be in a routine blood test.

The diagnosis of prediabetes is made the same way that a diagnosis of diabetes is made: by doing a blood glucose test in the laboratory. The critical *values* (numbers) in the test results are as follows:

- ✔ A normal fasting blood glucose result is less than 100 mg/dl (5.6 mmol/L).
- ✔ Prediabetes is diagnosed when the fasting blood glucose is between 100 and 125 mg/dl (5.6–6.9 mmol/L) on more than one occasion.

✔ Diabetes is diagnosed when the fasting blood glucose is 126 mg/dl (7 mmol/L) or greater on more than one occasion.

✔ A normal blood glucose level two hours after eating 75 grams of glucose is less than 140 mg/dl (7.8 mmol/L).

✔ Prediabetes is diagnosed when the glucose two hours after eating 75 grams of glucose is between 140 and 199 mg/dl (7.8–11.1 mmol/L) on more than one occasion.

✔ Diabetes is diagnosed when the glucose two hours after eating 75 grams of glucose is 200 mg/dl (11.1 mmol/L) or greater on more than one occasion.

Table 1-1 is a summary of these values.

Table 1-1	Normal, Prediabetic, and Diabetic Glucose Values		
Type of Test	*Normal*	*Prediabetes*	*Diabetes*
Fasting blood glucose	Less than 100 mg/dl	100–125 mg/dl	126 mg/dl or greater
Blood glucose two hours after eating 75 grams of glucose	Less than 140 mg/dl	140–199 mg/dl	200 mg/dl or greater

Here's what I can hear you saying: "You mean if my blood glucose is 99 mg/dl after fasting I don't have prediabetes, but if my blood glucose is 100 mg/dl — one measly milligram of glucose more — I do?" I'm afraid so.

These definitions are arbitrary. They have changed in the past, and they may do so again depending on scientific studies. For example, a fasting glucose result of greater than 140 mg/dl (7.8 mmol/L) used to be the cutoff point for a diagnosis of diabetes. Then doctors discovered that people who had fasting glucose levels below 140 mg/dl suffered from the complications of diabetes without having a diagnosis of diabetes. So they lowered the level for the diagnosis to 126 mg/dl (7 mmol/ L). Unfortunately, even some people with fasting blood glucose levels below 126 have shown up with complications of diabetes.

You should be familiar with some other terms for these levels of blood glucose, because you will likely read or hear about them:

✔ *Impaired fasting glucose* (IFG) is another name for the condition where the fasting blood glucose is between 100 and 125 mg/dl (5.6–6.9 mmol/L) after an overnight fast.

✔ *Impaired glucose tolerance* (IGT) is another name for the condition where the blood glucose is between 140 and 199 mg/dl (7.8–11.1 mmol/L) two hours after eating 75 grams of glucose.

Some people have impaired fasting glucose, while others have impaired glucose tolerance. Still others have both conditions combined, so the total number of people with prediabetes is *not* the sum of the people with IFG plus the people with IGT.

Other terms that you may hear should be disregarded because they have no clear meaning and are no longer used scientifically. These include:

✔ Borderline diabetes

✔ Touch of sugar

(It's important to get your terms straight. Otherwise, you may create confusion similar to what happened when a famous pianist told his audience that he was going to play a piece by a Danish composer named Mozart: Hans Christian Mozart.)

Someday it may be possible to make a diagnosis of prediabetes and diabetes without obtaining a blood sample by way of a needle stuck into a vein. A study by Melinda Sheffield-Moore, PhD, and others published in the March 2009 issue of *Diabetes Care* described a novel method to accomplish a diagnosis. People were given glucose to drink in which the carbon atoms were replaced by a harmless *radioisotope* (a form of the carbon that is made radioactive). The researchers found that the amount of radioactivity in the breath of people with prediabetes or diabetes was significantly lower than that in the breath of people with normal glucose tolerance. This result is expected because glucose is broken down for energy fairly quickly in healthy people, more slowly in people with prediabetes, and even more slowly in diabetics.

Focusing on type 2 prediabetes

There are two major types of diabetes called *type 1 diabetes mellitus* (T1DM) and *type 2 diabetes mellitus* (T2DM). (If you want to find out exactly what distinguishes them, pick up my book *Diabetes For Dummies,* which is also published by Wiley.) Here's a grossly oversimplified overview:

✔ Type 1 is an autoimmune disease that usually occurs in children.

✔ Type 2 may occur in either children or adults and is often associated with risk factors such as being overweight, having high blood pressure, and leading a sedentary lifestyle.

Prediabetes that can lead to type 1 diabetes is pretty similar to prediabetes that can lead to type 2 diabetes. However, in this book I focus on the prediabetes associated with type 2. When diabetes develops in type 1, it's because of a lack of the key hormone that controls blood glucose: *insulin* (see Chapter 2).

When diabetes develops in type 2, the body still has plenty of insulin but not enough to keep the blood glucose in the normal range because the body resists the action of insulin.

The word *prediabetes* in this book refers to the period between normal blood glucose control and type 2 diabetes.

Knowing the Recent History of Prediabetes

In this section, I discuss the reason for the development of the term *prediabetes*, as well as the fact that prediabetes is not an entirely benign condition.

Needing new language

The term *prediabetes* hasn't been around long. In fact, it was first used in 2002. It was introduced by the American Diabetes Association (ADA) and by then–Health and Human Services Secretary Tommy G. Thompson.

There were a number of reasons for the introduction of this term:

✔ The terms *impaired fasting glucose* and *impaired glucose tolerance* were meaningless to patients and required a lot of explaining.

✔ Other terms, like *touch of sugar* and *borderline diabetes,* were generally meaningless.

✔ Studies such as the Diabetes Prevention Program showed that diet and exercise resulting in a weight loss as little as 5 to 7 percent of someone's initial weight would lower the incidence of type 2 diabetes by up to 58 percent.

✔ A broadly understandable term was needed so that patients could know where they were and where they had to go with respect to diabetes. These people stood to benefit from lifestyle modification and other treatments.

Studies at the time showed that most people with prediabetes would go on to develop diabetes within ten years unless they made relatively modest changes in diet and exercise. Therefore, the ADA and Secretary Thompson put together an expert panel of doctors and other diabetes experts. The panel report stated that intervention in prediabetes is critical for three reasons:

✓ Just having glucose levels in the prediabetic range puts a person at a 50 percent greater risk of a heart attack or stroke.

✓ The development of type 2 diabetes can be delayed or prevented by modest lifestyle change.

✓ For many people, modest changes in lifestyle can turn back the clock and return elevated blood glucose levels to normal.

Along with the new term, the ADA recommended that physicians begin to screen their patients for prediabetes at age 45. Screening was especially important for people who answered yes to these questions:

✓ Do you have a relative with type 2 diabetes or heart disease?

✓ Are you overweight or obese?

✓ Do you have high blood pressure?

✓ Do you have a sedentary lifestyle?

✓ Do you have high levels of triglycerides and/or low levels of HDL cholesterol (both being types of fats measured in a blood test)?

✓ Do you belong to a higher-risk ethnic group, such as African American, Latino, or Asian American/Pacific Islander?

✓ Do you have apple-shaped rather than pear-shaped weight distribution? This means your excess weight is around your stomach rather than your hips.

✓ For women who have had children, did you develop diabetes during the pregnancy or have a baby who weighed more than 9 pounds at birth?

✓ For women, is there a history of *polycystic ovarian syndrome,* a condition that may include lack of periods, infertility, and increased hair on the body?

These days, if you can answer no to all these questions, you may be from outer space. So most doctors just screen all people over age 45.

Maria Sanchez was a 48-year-old woman whose mother had type 2 diabetes. Maria had a body mass index (BMI) of 31, which put her in the category of obese. (As I explain in Chapter 2, BMI shows how your weight relates to your height.) Her blood pressure was high at 150/94. She was from Nicaragua. Her body shape had the appearance of an apple, not a pear. She had had a baby who was 9 pounds, 4 ounces at birth. When she was tested for prediabetes, guess what? She didn't have it. Fooled you! But seriously, you can't make assumptions. That's why we have to test.

Understanding the risks

Prediabetes may not be associated with most of the problems of diabetes (which I discuss in Part IV), but your body is developing some reversible damage if you have this condition. I discuss the most important issues here.

Heart attacks and strokes

Numerous studies, including one in the journal *Circulation* in July 2007 and another in the *American Heart Journal* in August 2003, have shown that increased risks of heart disease and stroke exist even when blood glucose levels are significantly below the current glucose levels necessary for a diagnosis of diabetes. These risks even extend into the levels considered normal (less than 100 mg/dl of glucose). The risk has been found to be as much as doubled for people with prediabetes compared to people in the normal range for glucose. When prediabetes becomes diabetes, the risk doubles again.

When prediabetes is reversed and you get back to normal glucose levels, your risk of heart disease and stroke is significantly reduced. So you should make every effort to achieve normal blood glucose levels.

Retinopathy

Retinopathy is an abnormality within the eyeball that is specifically associated with diabetes; I describe it fully in Chapter 13. A study in the journal *Lancet* in March 2008 showed that retinopathy occurs even in the prediabetic state. As glucose levels increase, the prevalence of retinopathy increases dramatically. Although there is no definite threshold below which you don't have to worry about retinopathy, the more normal the blood glucose, the lower the risk for this complication.

Alzheimer's disease

Strong evidence exists that links diabetes to Alzheimer's disease. In fact, being diabetic *doubles* the odds of developing Alzheimer's disease. And even people with prediabetes show evidence of memory loss and *dementia* (loss of intellectual capacity).

A study in *Neurology* in August 2004 found that women with the highest levels of glucose (in the diabetes range) did worst on tests of mental capacity. Women in the prediabetic range did better, while women in the normal range did best.

I'm reminded of the story of the musician who told his wife at the airport that he wished he had brought his piano. "Why would you bring your piano to the airport?" inquired his wife. "Because I left the airline tickets on the piano," he replied.

Quality of life

At a conference in Uruguay in 2008, Consumer Health Sciences, an international provider of consumer information, presented data concerning the quality of life for the person with prediabetes. The data showed that a prediabetic's health-related quality of life is significantly lower than that of a healthy person. For example, someone with prediabetes loses an average of 5.6 weeks of work productivity per year compared to a healthy person.

Even though prediabetes is not as serious as diabetes, it does involve medical deterioration. The longer you allow yourself to have prediabetes, the greater the damage. Start to reverse it now!

Realizing Who Is Affected

Some groups of people are affected by prediabetes more than others, and they may even be affected when their blood glucose levels are lower than the levels that currently define prediabetes. (In the earlier section "Going from normal to prediabetes," I spell out those levels.)

As I write these words, studies are taking place to try to understand who may need to worry about prediabetes more than others. In addition, unfortunately, type 2 diabetes has begun to be found in children to a much greater extent than ever before, so many children are obviously going through a stage of prediabetes. And the largest group with prediabetes is the elderly. These age groups have special considerations that I introduce here and address in much more detail in Chapter 11.

Comparing ethnic groups

The prevalence of diabetes and prediabetes in non-Hispanic whites, non-Hispanic blacks, and Mexican Americans was last compared in 2005–2006 and published in *Diabetes Care* in February 2009. The study showed the expected increase in prediabetes with aging. While only 16 percent of people age 12 to 19 had prediabetes, 48 percent of people older than 75 had prediabetes. Table 1-2 shows the prevalence of prediabetes in the various ethnic groups over the age of 20.

Table 1-2	Prediabetes and Diabetes in Different Ethnic Groups	
Group	*Prediabetes*	*Diabetes*
Non-Hispanic white	29%	12%
Non-Hispanic black	25%	17%
Mexican Americans	32%	14%

Although the percent of Mexican Americans appears larger than the other groups with prediabetes, the authors of the study state that there is no significant difference among the groups. But when it comes to moving on to diabetes, minorities have significantly higher rates than whites.

Overall, the study showed that in 2005–2006, 13 percent of the adult U.S. population 20 years of age or older had diabetes (7.7 percent diagnosed and 5.3 percent undiagnosed), and another 29 percent had prediabetes. This means that more than *40 percent* of the U.S. population has a condition of high blood glucose.

The study compared glucose levels in the various populations in the years 1988–1994 with the 2005–2006 results. Surprisingly, the prevalence of prediabetes didn't change between the two time periods. However, the prevalence of diabetes was much higher in the later study. In 1988–1994, 9.3 percent of the U.S. population had diabetes (5.1 percent diagnosed and 4.2 percent undiagnosed). The group that showed the largest increase in diabetes between the two periods was non-Hispanic blacks.

Another ethnic group that shows a high rate of diabetes is Asian Americans. The prevalence of diagnosed diabetes in this group is 7.5 percent. The prevalence of prediabetes in Asian Americans is not known.

The enormous increase in cases of high glucose has resulted in a correspondingly huge increase in the cost of care, which I discuss in the last part of this chapter.

Considering children and adolescents

By the end of 2007, the Centers for Disease Control and the National Institutes of Health were reporting that 2 million U.S. children and adolescents had prediabetes. The numbers have increased since then. The reason for all this prediabetes in children is the growing epidemic of obesity in children.

The prevalence of obesity among children ages 6 to 11 more than doubled in the past two decades, going from 6.5 percent in 1980 to 17 percent in 2006. Among adolescents ages 12 to 19, obesity has tripled in that time frame, going from 5 percent to 17.6 percent.

Not only are children with obesity at greater risk for prediabetes and diabetes, but they may suffer bone and joint problems, *sleep apnea* (periods of stopping breathing during sleep that lead to extreme fatigue during the day), and social and psychological problems. In Chapter 11, I offer specific advice about prediabetes and obesity in children and adolescents.

Finding rampant prediabetes in the elderly

The elderly (which means people who are older than me) are at the greatest risk of developing prediabetes and diabetes. About one-third of people age 65 and older have diabetes, and another 30 percent have prediabetes. Only one-third of elderly people have neither condition. When these conditions are combined with the other ills common to the elderly, such as heart disease, reduced kidney function, and mental deterioration, the results are significant sickness, the need for many types of medications, and complications that require a lot of medical care.

In the elderly, using just the fasting blood glucose test to diagnose prediabetes misses most of the cases. To really determine the prevalence of prediabetes in this group, taking a glucose reading two hours after drinking 75 grams of glucose is necessary.

Because it's such a complicated problem, prediabetes in the elderly deserves its own large section in Chapter 11.

Prediabetes in the elderly is reversible just as it is in children, adolescents, and adults. Reversing the condition may be more difficult because of the reduced ability to exercise and the tendency to eat a less healthful diet, but it's never too late to prevent and reverse prediabetes.

Considering the Costs

All this potential sickness and real sickness comes with very large costs. In 2008, the cost for diabetes and prediabetes in the United States was determined to be $218 billion. One of every ten dollars spent for health care was spent for these conditions. That number was up from $173 billion in 2007, and it's not likely to go down anytime soon. In this section, I discuss both the dollar costs and the other costs of prediabetes.

Actual health costs

Most of the costs of diabetes and prediabetes are for treating the complications that I discuss in Part IV. These complications include

- Eye disease possibly leading to blindness
- Kidney disease possibly leading to kidney failure
- Nerve disease possibly leading to severe pain or amputation
- Heart disease and arterial disease possibly leading to heart attacks, strokes, or severe leg pain

The fact is that the top three complications will *never occur* if prediabetes is reversed or never allowed to occur in the first place. Stopping prediabetes in its tracks is preventive medicine. Unfortunately, health insurance companies are willing to spend the thousands needed for treating the end results of disease but won't spend the much smaller sums needed to prevent the complications in the first place.

The Diabetes Prevention Program showed that preventive methods like diet and exercise delay the development of type 2 diabetes by an average of 11 years and reduce the number of new cases of diabetes by 20 percent. The costs for time with doctors and medications could be reduced by $1,100 per year per person.

Other economic costs

As I write these words in mid-2009, with the economy of the United States and the rest of the world in a very precarious position, the huge costs of medical care are a major drain on our society. The automobile industry is the best-known example of an industry that has been hugely affected by health-care costs for its workers, much of those costs generated by diabetes and prediabetes.

The Diabetes Prevention Program showed that prevention of diabetes would save $8,800 of societal costs per person. *Societal costs* are the indirect costs like lost productivity, taxes paid for health care and disability, and other non-medical costs.

Social costs

People who suffer blindness or kidney failure can't work at the level of people without these conditions, so much of their productivity is lost. Sometimes these complications — and the heart disease that is so much worse with diabetes — lead to an early death, so the losses from diabetes also affect entire families.

Because prediabetes and type 2 diabetes are now being seen so often in children and adolescents, we can expect that people will develop complications at much younger ages. People who should be in the prime of their lives will instead be suffering illness and premature death.

The goal of this book is to show you that such a path isn't inevitable and that these costs can be avoided. Turn the page to begin finding out how to walk the road back to health.

Chapter 2

Suspecting Prediabetes in Yourself or a Loved One

*Y*ou've gained a few pounds over the years. You don't have the energy you used to have. Your mother has diabetes, and you have been reading about this condition called prediabetes so you want to know whether you may have it. In this chapter you find everything you need to know to tell whether you or a loved one may have prediabetes or diabetes. If, after reading this chapter, your suspicion is confirmed, the next step is to see a doctor to get yourself tested.

Taking a Risk Quiz

Dr. Richelle Koopman and others at the University of Missouri have developed a clinical tool that you can use to assess the chance that a *fasting blood glucose test* (a test that screens for prediabetes — see Chapter 10) will come back abnormal. They published a paper in the November/December 2008 issue of the *Annals of Family Medicine*.

The tool focuses on six characteristics that are most important in determining your susceptibility to prediabetes and diabetes:

✔ Age
✔ Sex
✔ Body mass index

 ✔ Family history of diabetes

 ✔ Heart rate

 ✔ High blood pressure

To determine your body mass index (BMI), multiply your weight in pounds by 703. Divide the result by your height in inches. Divide that result by your height in inches again. (If you happen to know your height in meters and your weight in kilograms, you can skip the first multiplication.)

Each characteristic is given a numerical value:

 ✔ Age: 20–27=1, 28–35=2, 36–44=3, 45–64=4

 ✔ Sex: Male=3, female=0

 ✔ Body mass index: Less than 25=0, 25–29.9=2, 30 or more=3

 ✔ Family history: No=0, yes=1

 ✔ Heart rate: Less than 70=0, 70–79=1, 80–89=2, 90–99=3, equal to or greater than 100=4

 ✔ High blood pressure: No=0, yes=1

High blood pressure refers to a reading of equal to or greater than 140/90. If either number is elevated consistently, you have high blood pressure.

The reason that the age categories stop at 64 is that the authors found the risk for all adults 65 and over was so high that they have a high risk of abnormal fasting blood glucose (an indicator of prediabetes) regardless of the other characteristics.

Consider an example of how to use this risk quiz: Sol is a 43-year-old man with a BMI of 28.6. No one in his family has had diabetes. His heart rate is 68, and his blood pressure is normal. He gets 3 points for age, 3 points for his gender, 2 points for BMI, no points for family history, no points for heart rate, and no points for blood pressure. His total is 8.

Here's how the University of Missouri researchers interpret the numerical results of this quiz:

 ✔ 5 means the likelihood of having an abnormal fasting blood glucose result is 1.53. This means that it is 1.53 times more likely that the patient has prediabetes than that the patient does not have prediabetes.

 ✔ 6 means the likelihood is 1.80.

 ✔ 7 means the likelihood is 2.16.

 ✔ 8 means the likelihood is 2.54.

 ✔ 9 means the likelihood is 3.26.

A result of 8, 9, or higher means it is highly likely that a fasting blood glucose test will be positive, indicating you have prediabetes.

Cholesterol levels are not used in this tool because they don't change the result. Resting heart rate is used instead of exercise history because it is much easier to measure and quantify.

Go ahead and figure out your own number. If it is 8 or above, visit your doctor so he can do a fasting blood glucose test. If you prefer to start lowering your number in the meantime, read Chapter 4.

Identifying Key Risk Factors That You Can Control

There's not much you can do about your age and your sex. (A sex-change operation won't help.) But you can alter all the other risk factors that promote prediabetes and diabetes. In this section, I introduce these factors and point you to the chapters later in the book that give specific advice on how to affect them.

Understanding the role of calories

A calorie is a calorie is a calorie. Whether calories come from protein, fat, or carbohydrate (the only known sources of calories), too many of them will make you overweight or obese, and too few of them will make you skinny. Despite the huge number of books that suggest you are better off on a low carbohydrate diet or a high protein diet or a high grapefruit diet or whatever, the truth is that when it comes to your weight, the *type* of food you eat doesn't matter.

The most definitive study that shows this fact was published in *The New England Journal of Medicine* in February 2009. A group of 811 overweight adults were randomly assigned to one of four diets that differed in the percent of calories from fat, protein, and carbohydrate. The total calories eaten were the same in all groups. The results were as follows:

- ✔ At six months of dieting, regardless of the diet, people had lost an average of 13 pounds.

- ✔ By 12 months, the participants started to regain their weight because they were not following the diet as carefully.

✔ At two years, weight loss was similar whether the participants were eating 15 percent protein or 25 percent protein, whether they were eating 20 percent fat or 40 percent fat, and whether they were eating 65 percent carbohydrate or 35 percent carbohydrate.

✔ Of those who completed the two years, the average weight loss was 9 pounds.

✔ Feelings of fullness, hunger, and satisfaction with the diet were the same for all the groups.

✔ Attendance at group and individual instructional sessions was strongly associated with weight loss.

✔ Cholesterol levels and blood glucose levels were improved to the same extent in all groups.

What more can I say? Does this mean that book writers will stop trying to convince us that no carbohydrates are better than no fat, or vice versa? Do cows really jump over the moon? If the shelves of bookstores were cleared of such books, there would be a lot of empty space.

Later in this book, I provide you with some delicious recipes that show you that you can eat great food and still follow a good diet. So long as you keep your total calories within the bounds that I suggest in Chapter 16, feel free to enjoy any of the recipes you find there.

Focusing on your weight

In the first section of this chapter, I explain that if you have a normal body mass index, which means your weight is appropriate for your height, it adds nothing to your chance of having an abnormal fasting blood glucose. If your BMI puts you in the overweight category (25–29.9), you have to add 2 to your total risk number. If you are obese (a BMI of 30 or more), you have to add 3. Obviously, weight adds a large contribution to the risk of prediabetes.

In Chapter 6, I provide a chart that you can use to determine your BMI. And there is another way to determine whether your weight is appropriate. Start with your height in inches. If you are female, give yourself 100 pounds for 5 feet (60 inches) plus 5 pounds for every inch over 5 feet. So if you are a female 5 feet 4 inches in height, your ideal weight is 120 pounds. Your correct weight range is 120 plus or minus 10 percent. So a 5'4" woman can weigh anywhere from 108 to 132 pounds and still be considered normal. At 108 pounds, this woman's BMI is 18.5. At 132 pounds, she has a BMI of 22.6, which is just right.

If you are a man, you get 106 pounds for 5 feet and 6 pounds for every inch over 5 feet. Say you are the same height as the woman above, 5'4". Your ideal weight is 130 pounds, and your range is 117 to 143 pounds. That gives a BMI of 20.6 to 24.5, which is just about perfect.

Getting down to these ideal weights is not necessary for your health. A weight loss of just 5 to 10 percent may be all you need to get your blood glucose, blood pressure, and cholesterol where they need to be. If you want to be a fashion model, that's up to you. I just want you to be a model of health.

One doctor I know suggested that his patient eat normally for two days and then skip a day. The patient came back after a month and had lost a lot of weight. He told the doctor that he almost died on the third day. The doctor asked, "From hunger?" He answered, "No, from skipping."

Getting up and moving

How much exercise is necessary for you? Chances are it is more than you are currently doing. It seems that every health organization wants to offer guidelines for physical activity, but two major sources just came out with their advice, which I discuss here. Following either one of these guidelines will provide all the exercise you need, not only to reverse prediabetes but also for good general health.

Following Health and Human Services guidelines

The U.S. Department of Health and Human Services issued its latest guidelines in 2008. The guidelines are based on the research of the Physical Activity Guidelines Advisory Committee, which found that:

- ✔ Regular physical activity lowers the risk for many adverse health outcomes.

- ✔ Although some physical activity is better than none, higher intensity, greater frequency, and/or longer duration of physical activity provide additional benefits for most health outcomes.

- ✔ At least 150 minutes per week of moderate-intensity physical activity, such as brisk walking, is needed for most health benefits, but more physical activity provides additional benefits.

- ✔ Aerobic (endurance) and muscle-strengthening (resistance) physical activity both promote better health.

- ✔ In every studied racial and ethnic group, and in children and adolescents, young and middle-aged adults, and older adults, physical activity is linked to health benefits.

✔ People with disabilities also receive health benefits from physical activity.

✔ The benefits provided by physical activity far outweigh the risks for harm.

The guidelines offer separate recommendations for children and adolescents and for adults, including older adults. Additional guidelines are provided for older adults.

Guidelines for children

✔ Children and adolescents should engage in at least one hour of physical activity daily, preferably in physical activities that are appropriate for their age, that are enjoyable, and that offer variety.

✔ Most of this activity should be either moderate or vigorous-intensity aerobic physical activity.

✔ Vigorous-intensity physical activity, muscle-strengthening physical activity, and bone-strengthening physical activity should be performed at least three days per week.

Guidelines for adults, including older adults

✔ All adults should avoid inactivity. Participation in any amount of physical activity is associated with some health benefits relative to no physical activity.

✔ At least 150 minutes per week of moderate-intensity or 75 minutes a week of vigorous-intensity aerobic physical activity, or an equivalent combination of moderate- and vigorous-intensity aerobic activity offers substantial health benefits.

✔ Aerobic activity should preferably be spread throughout the week and performed in episodes of at least 10 minutes.

✔ Aerobic physical activity of 300 minutes per week of moderate intensity, or 150 minutes per week of vigorous intensity, or an equivalent combination of moderate- and vigorous-intensity activity is associated with additional and more extensive health benefits.

✔ Engaging in physical activity beyond this amount provides additional health benefits.

✔ Muscle-strengthening activities that are moderate or high intensity and involve all major muscle groups should be performed on two or more days per week for additional health benefits.

Additional guidelines specific to older adults

✔ When chronic conditions prevent older adults from doing 150 minutes of moderate-intensity aerobic activity per week, they should be as physically active as their abilities and conditions allow. They should understand whether and how their conditions affect their ability to do regular physical activity safely.

- ✔ Older adults at risk of falling should do exercises that maintain or improve balance.

- ✔ Older adults should determine their level of effort for physical activity relative to their fitness level.

Adhering to American College of Sports Medicine guidelines

The American College of Sports Medicine (ACSM) updated its guidelines in 2009. They state that "the purpose of the current update was to focus on new information that has been published after 1999, which may indicate that increased levels of physical activity may be necessary for prevention of weight gain, for weight loss and prevention of weight regain compared to those recommended in the 2001 position stand."

ACSM defines its guidelines in terms of *metabolic equivalents* (METs). One MET is the energy (oxygen) used by the body at rest, while sitting quietly or reading a book. The harder your body works during the activity, the more oxygen is consumed and the higher the MET level. The different levels of intensity of activity are

- ✔ Light-intensity activity, which results in no increase in breathing or heart rate.

- ✔ Moderate-intensity activity, which burns 3 to 6 METs. It causes an increase in breathing and/or heart rate and burns 3.5 to 7 kilocalories per minute. You are sweating but can still carry on a conversation.

- ✔ Vigorous-intensity activity, which burns more than 6 METs per minute. It causes rapid breathing and a substantial increase in heart rate and burns more than 7 kilocalories per minute. Jogging is an example. It is difficult to carry on a conversation.

The ACSM's recommendations are for all healthy adults aged 18 to 65. They suggest that you

- ✔ Do moderately intense aerobic exercise 30 minutes five days a week or do vigorously intense exercise 20 minutes five days a week.

- ✔ Do eight to ten strength training (resistance) exercises, with eight to twelve repetitions of each exercise, twice a week.

Chapters 7 and 17 provide specific ways that you can meet these recommendations.

The most common excuse that I get from my patients for not doing the recommended amount of exercise is lack of time. If you notice in the above recommendations, you can substitute 20 minutes of vigorous activity for 30 minutes of moderately intense exercise. Recent research suggests that it may be possible to obtain significant health benefits from even less time.

A study in the January 2009 issue of *BMC Endocrine Disorders* provides some amazing information. The title of the study is "Extremely short duration of high intensity interval training substantially improves insulin action in young healthy males." The men in the study performed a total of 15 minutes of supervised cycle sprints over two weeks. They did six sessions over the two weeks. Each session consisted of four to six 30-second cycle sprints. No session, therefore, lasted longer than three minutes.

It had already been shown that such exercise produces improvement in aerobic function. In this study, the authors showed that there was improvement in sensitivity to insulin and a lowering of the blood glucose. Now tell me you don't have 15 minutes every two weeks to spare for your health!

Dealing with stress

Stress plays an important role in both prediabetes and diabetes. Some people respond to stress with great agitation, while others find a way to cope with the stress in a more relaxed way. Your body secretes *stress hormones:* chemicals that help you to respond to stress. For example, your body may make a lot of adrenaline, which increases your strength, makes you more awake, and allows you to fight or flee more effectively. Unfortunately, as a side effect, the stress hormones raise your blood glucose.

The other major effect of stress is the tendency to stop doing the things that make you healthy. When someone is sick in the family or you lose a job, your first priority is not to get the exercise you need or to stick to the correct daily level of calories. You have other things on your mind. Your health may suffer as a result.

In Chapter 8, I offer a detailed program for dealing with the effects of stress. One great suggestion is to try to deal with it through humor. Obviously, the use of humor depends on the source of the stress. It would be hard to find humor in a death in the family, but many of my patients with diabetes have been able to find humor in their condition. They tend to do better when they can. If you don't believe me, read Norman Cousins' book *Anatomy of an Illness as Perceived by the Patient* (W.W. Norton & Co.). He was able to cure a fatal disease by surrounding himself with things that made him laugh: movies, cartoons, CDs of his favorite comedians, and so forth.

One of my favorite quotes comes from Joel Goodman of the Humor Project: "Someday we will laugh at this, why not now!" Of course, someone has also said, "If laughter were really the best medicine, doctors would have found a way to charge for it."

Understanding How Prediabetes and Diabetes Develop

When your metabolism is normal, your blood glucose is controlled within a narrow range, from a low of about 70 mg/dl (3.9 mmol/L) when you are fasting to a high of about 139 mg/dl (7.7 mmol/L) one hour after eating. This section explains how a healthy body keeps such a tight grip on glucose and what goes wrong when that grip slips.

Keeping glucose under control

Insulin is a *hormone* (a chemical made in an organ, in this case the pancreas) that enters the blood stream and affects cells throughout the body. Insulin opens these cells so glucose can enter and provide the energy needed by your muscles, your fat, and many other tissues. Without insulin, glucose in your blood stream can't be utilized.

Insulin permits the building up of muscle, fat, and other tissues. In this sense it is the builder hormone. You can't build your body without insulin. It also provides for storage of excess glucose in the form of glycogen so that it is ready to quickly provide energy as the glucose level falls. You do not live long without insulin.

Losing control of glucose

Your blood glucose begins to rise if you are lacking sufficient insulin or if the insulin in your body is not working effectively. The latter situation is called *insulin resistance.* When the glucose rises to 180 mg/dl (10 mmol/L) in the blood, your kidneys can no longer return all the glucose to the blood and it starts to spill into your urine. You begin to develop some annoying complications. Because the glucose in prediabetes can rise as high as 199 mg/dl, you can have these complications even in prediabetes. They include

- ✔ Frequent urination and thirst because the glucose in the urine pulls water out of your body and fills your bladder, making you want to urinate more often. As you lose water you get thirsty.

- ✔ Fatigue because the cells are not getting the energy they need.

- ✔ Persistent vaginal infection in women because there is some spilling of glucose over the vaginal tissues, and yeast loves a sweet surface to grow on. There is itching, burning, an abnormal discharge, and sometimes an odor.

I say much more about short-term complications in Chapter 12.

As the insulin in your body declines further or becomes even less effective, you start to develop long-term complications, especially heart disease, eye disease, kidney disease, and nerve disease. At this point you have diabetes. You can still prevent these unpleasant complications by lifestyle changes and perhaps medication, but isn't it so much better never to get to this stage?

Chapter 13 tells you all you need to know about the potential long-term complications of diabetes.

Seeking a Medical Diagnosis

Earlier in this chapter I provide a risk quiz that you can take if you think you may have prediabetes. Obviously, the quiz can leave you with a large amount of suspicion but not a definite diagnosis. For a diagnosis, you need to see a doctor.

Does that doctor have to be a specialist? The answer is no. A good *internist* (a general doctor who takes care of adults but does not do surgery) or even a family physician is the right person to go to at the start to make the diagnosis. After the diagnosis of prediabetes is made, you can decide if this doctor is the right person to stay with to get the help you need to reverse the condition. If not, you want to see a specialist. In this section, I offer advice for finding both kinds of physicians.

Choosing a general doctor

There are numerous ways to choose a general doctor. Don't make this decision lightly. Remember that this person will take care of all your medical problems and even some of your psychological problems.

Depending upon your situation, one or another of the following scenarios may work for you:

- ✔ **Using a recommendation from a friend or a family member that you trust:** This is often the best source for locating an excellent general doctor.

- ✔ **Selecting from a list provided by your health insurance company:** Your insurance provider may require this step. The screening done by these companies before they sign up doctors is often minimal, but you will do the final screening in any case.

✔ **Contacting your local medical society:** It can provide a list of qualified general physicians from which you, again, will do the ultimate screening. Remember that the medical society will accept any doctor with an MD after his name.

✔ **Contacting the department of medicine of a local medical center or medical school:** The doctors that they recommend are generally highly qualified but may be more immersed in research than patient care.

✔ **Checking out ratings in newspapers and magazines or on the Internet:** Your own local magazine may feature such ratings. My local magazine recently featured an article called "Top Bay Area Physicians," for example. If you use this source, check out how the doctors are rated: by other physicians, by patients, or by nurses. Each group of raters looks at doctors from a different perspective.

Doing your research

If all you know is a doctor's name, you can't assume that you've found the right person. And if you have more than one name to choose from, how do you choose the right one? You have to do some research, both before you get to the doctor's office and after you are there.

Before you see the doctor

There are several ways to check the doctor's credentials before you arrive:

✔ **Check the Web site of your state's medical board.** You can start at the Web site of the Federation of State Medical Boards: www.fsmb.org. Click on "Member Services" on the home page, and choose "Directory of State Medical Boards." Find your state's medical board from that list. You should be able to enter the doctor's name to find out if he has ever been disciplined for an infraction of medical care or if he has lost a malpractice suit. For example, my own state, California, has a choice on its first page, "Check Your Doctor, click here." When you do, it tells you what kind of information to expect, from medical wrongdoing to disciplines in other states to hospital disciplines to malpractice suits where the settlement is greater than $30,000. The Web site *will not* tell you of complaints made to the board, investigations that did not result in discipline, or pending or dismissed malpractice cases.

Go ahead: Visit the California site and put in my name. You'll find that my license is renewed and current and that I have a clean slate!

✔ **Find out from the doctor's office where he was trained.** Make sure that the medical school is in the United States. If not, make sure he trained in a country whose medical standards are accredited by the National Committee on Foreign Medical Education and Accreditation at www.ed.gov/about/bdscomm/list/ncfmea.html. This U.S. government organization does not review individual medical schools — only the standards that a foreign country establishes for its medical schools to see whether they are comparable to U.S. standards.

✔ **Find out how much time he sets aside for patients.** Your first visit should last 45 minutes to one hour. Return visits should last at least 15 minutes.

✔ **Try to find out how long he keeps his patients waiting.** Your time is valuable. Waiting in the doctor's office for an hour is no pleasure — especially if half his other patients are coughing on you — unless you really want to catch up on your latest magazine reading. (The magazines are probably old anyway.)

✔ **Check out the receptionist on the phone.** If the receptionist is friendly and helpful, that's a major plus, because you will be dealing with her any time you want to reach the doctor or have a billing question.

At the doctor's office

There are plenty of ways to judge a doctor both before and when you see her. Look for some of the following clues:

✔ Is the office generally neat and well-maintained?

✔ Do other patients have positive things to say about this doctor?

✔ Do the receptionist and/or nurses appear happy to be working there and greet you with a friendly smile?

✔ How long do you have to wait before finally seeing the doctor?

✔ Does the doctor look you straight in the eyes?

✔ Does she spend enough time with you?

✔ Do you get all your questions answered?

✔ Does she seem to have a genuine interest in your problems?

✔ Does she use e-mail to inform you of test results or promise to call if she doesn't use e-mail? Does she keep this promise?

Even if your experience is wholly positive, your general physician still may not be the right one to take you through the major lifestyle changes required when you have prediabetes. With a diagnosis in hand, you may consider a specialist.

Choosing a specialist

Most of the techniques in the section on choosing a general doctor are applicable to choosing a specialist, but there are specialist societies that you should know about to help you in your choice. All of the societies I list here can be reached through my Web site: www.drrubin.com. On the main page, look for "Related Websites." Click on "Diabetes" for the American Diabetes Association and "Thyroid" for all the rest.

American Diabetes Association

This major organization, found at www.diabetes.org, can offer a lot of advice about choosing a doctor. From the main page, choose "All About Diabetes" on the left, then "Who's On Your Health Care Team?" From there you can choose the person you are looking for, whether a doctor, a diabetes educator, a dietitian, or a social worker, and learn both how to select one and what services to expect from each one. This site does not offer a way to select an individual physician, however.

American Association of Clinical Endocrinologists

Go to www.aace.com to reach this organization, or click through my Web site. On the left side of the first page, find the list "For Public" and click on "Find an Endocrinologist." This takes you to the "AACE Physician Finder." Select U.S. or Other. Assuming that you select U.S., the city, state, ZIP, and *radius* (the distance from that ZIP that you are willing to travel) will pop up, along with Specialty. Fill in those boxes. You will receive a list of specialists in alphabetical order who are within that distance from that ZIP code. The site even provides interest areas for some of the doctors so you can make sure that diabetes mellitus is on the list, unless you filled in that term in the Specialty box already.

Endocrine Society

You can find this organization at www.endo-society.org or by clicking on my Web site. At the lower right of the home page, click on "The Hormone Foundation" to find physician referrals. On the left side of that page, fill in your ZIP code and choose the Search Area. If you filled in my ZIP, you would find a list sorted by the distance from that ZIP. Of course, my name would be at the top of the list, but you would also find 21 matches in case you don't like me.

Making sure your doctor covers the bases

So you are satisfied that you have found the right person at last (sigh!). If he is the right doctor, he will know what to do to find out if you have prediabetes. A number of tests and procedures need to be done at your first visit. I discuss them at length in Chapter 10, including how to interpret them. Here I want to just list them so you make sure all the important areas are covered. They include:

✔ **Fasting blood glucose or blood glucose two hours after drinking 75 grams of glucose:** The first test is usually the one that's done because it is so much simpler, but it depends on the doctor. Remember to ask that the test be done again if the first one is abnormal. You don't want to make a diagnosis of prediabetes or diabetes based on a single test.

✔ **Your weight, height, and body mass index:** This information serves as a baseline and allows the doctor to set a goal for your weight.

✔ **Your blood pressure:** High blood pressure is a major contributor to the complications that develop in diabetes as well as prediabetes.

✔ **Your lipid profile:** This test includes your total cholesterol, your *LDL* or bad cholesterol, your *HDL* or good cholesterol, and your triglycerides. This test must be done after an overnight fast — the same as the fasting blood glucose.

✔ **Kidney tests:** These include a urine test to see whether there is a tiny but abnormal amount of protein in your urine, which would suggest the beginning of kidney damage, and blood tests to see whether your body is getting rid of wastes in a proper manner. These tests include a blood urea nitrogen (BUN) and creatinine.

The doctor will recommend other tests if any of these are abnormal, including an eye examination by an eye doctor or optometrist, a foot examination, and so forth. I get into the nitty gritty of these follow-ups in Chapter 10.

Chapter 3

Tracking the Transition from Prediabetes to Diabetes

*M*edically speaking, the distinction between prediabetes and diabetes is designated by going from one level of blood glucose to another. But in real life, the division between the two conditions is not so sharp. People with blood glucose levels that are persistently high but not quite in the diabetic range sometimes have complications that are supposed to be found only in diabetes, like eye disease and nerve disease. (So your goal should be not only to avoid going from prediabetes to diabetes but also to keep your blood glucose in the normal range.)

The bottom line: The risk of getting diabetes is as much as ten times greater if you have prediabetes than if you have normal blood glucose levels. So if you suspect you have prediabetes, you need to act now to make sure it doesn't become diabetes. In this chapter, I explain why you don't want diabetes to happen to you.

I start the chapter by talking about the signs and symptoms that should alert you that you may be making the transition into diabetes. I then introduce the short-term and long-term complications that arise when you become a person with diabetes. These complications get more detailed attention in Part IV, but here I just want you to understand what you are up against if you permit the transition to take place.

With rare exceptions, you *can* prevent the transition from prediabetes to diabetes.

Turning Prediabetes into Diabetes

In the effort to prevent prediabetes from turning into diabetes, doctors and patients hit a number of roadblocks:

 ✔ Health insurance companies don't usually pay for treatments to improve lifestyle.

 ✔ No FDA-approved medications exist for treating impaired fasting glucose or impaired glucose tolerance (conditions that I define in Chapter 1).

 ✔ Doctors don't share a unanimous approach to treating prediabetes.

 ✔ There are no definite goals as to levels of weight, blood glucose, blood pressure, or blood cholesterol that are necessary to prevent diabetes.

We have to pressure health insurance companies to encourage lifestyle change by paying for the people who facilitate it, such as dietitians, physical trainers, psychologists, and social workers. We have to encourage the FDA to approve medications or even surgery (see Chapter 19) for prediabetes if lifestyle change does not work. And we have to set some kind of goal, even if it's an approximation, for weight, blood glucose, blood pressure, and cholesterol levels.

But while we work on tearing down these roadblocks, people continue to make the transition from prediabetes to diabetes every day. How do you know when you've crossed the line?

In Chapter 1, I explain that when the result of a fasting blood glucose test is 126 mg/dl (7 mmol/L) or greater, or when your blood glucose two hours after consuming 75 grams of glucose is greater than or equal to 200 mg/dl (11.1 mmol/L) on two occasions, a diagnosis of diabetes is made. That's how the lab decides that you've transitioned into diabetes.

But before you even go to the doctor and have a blood test, you can look for these clues that you're crossing the line:

 ✔ You are gaining weight.

 ✔ You have decreased your level of exercise or are injured and can't exercise.

 ✔ You urinate frequently and often feel thirsty.

 ✔ You feel fatigued.

 ✔ You are a woman who is getting frequent vaginal infections with yeast or some other organism.

So what actually happens to tip prediabetes into diabetes? Nothing very earth-shaking. Just getting a little older can lower your insulin sensitivity so that your body's insulin can't keep your fasting glucose level under 126 mg/dl.

Or allowing yourself to gain a few pounds can do it. Reducing your physical activity can result in a rise in your blood glucose to 126 mg/dl or higher, especially if you were doing vigorous physical exercise before and can't now because of an injury or illness. If several of these things are happening at the same time, which is often the case, the likelihood that prediabetes will turn into diabetes is even greater.

People with either impaired fasting glucose or impaired glucose tolerance (see Chapter 1) convert to diabetes at the rate of about 8 to 10 percent per year. However, for people who have *both* conditions, the rate is much higher.

Recognizing Short-term Effects of Diabetes

Symptoms that develop when diabetes occurs are divided into short-term and long-term complications. I discuss them at length in Chapters 12 through 14, but in this chapter I offer an overview so you know what you're trying to avoid.

Short-term effects result from persistent elevations of blood glucose or sudden falls in blood glucose. They are immediately treatable, and the abnormality is reversed as long as the rise or fall in blood glucose doesn't recur. These short-term complications can occur at any stage in the course of diabetes, not just at the beginning. But as patients become more familiar with their disease, these effects usually occur less often.

Handling hypoglycemia

Hypoglycemia means low blood glucose. There is no exact level of blood glucose that defines hypoglycemia because some people develop symptoms at 70 mg/dl (3.9 mmol/L) and others are still comfortable at that blood level but have symptoms at 60 mg/dl (3.3 mmol/L). Hypoglycemia does not result from the diabetes itself but from the drugs that we use to treat high blood glucose.

Symptoms
Some of the important symptoms that suggest hypoglycemia are

- ✔ Hunger
- ✔ Sweating
- ✔ Mental confusion or even coma

- ✔ Rapid heartbeat
- ✔ Headache
- ✔ Visual disturbances like double vision

One of my patients with diabetes had to get to an appointment. She had taken her diabetes medication but couldn't stop to eat. She got into her car and was spotted weaving back and forth across the lanes of traffic. A policeman stopped her and concluded that she was drunk. She was unable to tell him that she had diabetes. At the jail someone noticed she was wearing a bracelet that said she was a person with diabetes. She was given a glass of orange juice and promptly recovered. Unfortunately, it took her quite a while to prove to the Department of Motor Vehicles that she could drive safely.

Triggers

Here are some of the substances and circumstances that can bring on hypoglycemia either by themselves or when you have taken a drug to lower your blood glucose:

- ✔ *Sulfonylureas,* which are drugs taken by mouth to lower glucose with names like Orinase, Diabinase, and glyburide
- ✔ Insulin, usually taken by injection
- ✔ Aspirin or other salicylates
- ✔ Alcohol
- ✔ Too little food for the glucose-lowering drug in your body
- ✔ Too much exercise for the glucose-lowering drug in your body

Simple treatments

Most hypoglycemia is mild and responds to simple measures. You should be better within 20 minutes after taking one these treatments:

- ✔ Two sugar cubes
- ✔ Two or three glucose tablets
- ✔ Six ounces of a sugary soft drink
- ✔ Eight ounces of milk
- ✔ Four ounces of orange juice

Managing ketoacidosis

Ketoacidosis isn't common in someone with type 2 diabetes, but it occasionally happens, especially when the person has a severe infection or great physical stress. What happens is that the blood glucose rises very high, sometimes to 500 or 600 mg/dl (27.8 to 33.3 mmol/L). No glucose is getting into cells so the body turns to fat for energy. As fat breaks down, it produces a lot of acidic breakdown products. The large amount of sugar in the blood can't be held back by the kidneys and flows into the urine, pulling a lot of body water with it. The person becomes dehydrated and *acidotic* (meaning she has an abnormal increase of acids in her blood), leading to nausea and vomiting, which further depletes the body not only of water but of minerals like potassium.

You may notice that you have some symptoms of ketoacidosis and begin to suspect that you have this complication. But that diagnosis is best made by a doctor, preferably in the hospital where you can begin treatment at once.

Symptoms

Ketoacidosis is associated with many symptoms, which make it fairly easy to realize what is happening. Among them are

- ✔ Nausea and vomiting.

- ✔ Rapid breathing known as *Kussmaul breathing*. Your body is attempting to reduce the acid in your blood by blowing it off through the lungs. Your breath has a fruity smell due to the acetone from the fat.

- ✔ Extreme tiredness and drowsiness because the blood that circulates in your brain is thick like syrup and is missing essential substances.

- ✔ Weakness due to lack of fuel (glucose), which is elevated in the blood but can't get into your cells.

Signs

Unlike symptoms, which you can notice yourself, *signs* are the things that are observed by other people, particularly your doctor when you reach the hospital. The signs of ketoacidosis are

- ✔ High blood glucose, usually more than 300 mg/dl (16.6 mmol/L)

- ✔ High levels of acid in your blood

- ✔ High levels of *ketones* (the products of the breakdown of fats) in your blood and urine

- ✔ Dry skin and tongue consistent with dehydration

- ✔ Deficiency of potassium in your body

- ✔ Acetone smell on your breath

There is another situation, when you aren't sick, which may cause you to have a lot of ketones in your blood and urine. That's when you go on a diet and your fat cells begin to break down. Your glucose levels are likely to be just fine in this situation.

Treatment

Treatment of ketoacidosis is done by a physician in the hospital. The doctor gives you insulin to make up for the lack of active insulin in your body, replaces lost potassium, and gives you a lot of intravenous fluids to rehydrate your body.

The treatments are all done very rapidly, and sometimes the patient is okay in 36 hours. However, if the ketoacidosis was brought on by a severe infection or other trauma, it may resist treatment and even end in death.

Dealing with the hyperosmolar syndrome

People who have this short-term complication of diabetes have some of the highest blood glucose levels. There is so much glucose in the blood that it is literally like maple syrup. As you can imagine, your blood vessels were not meant to carry maple syrup.

This complication often occurs in elderly people who were not even known to have diabetes. They may be at home or in a nursing home where they are not carefully monitored, and they become dehydrated. If they develop nausea, vomiting, or diarrhea, they may end up with even more dehydration.

The elderly also have reduced kidney function. While a younger kidney begins to leak glucose into the urine and thus outside the body at a blood level of 180 mg/dl (10 mmol/L), the older kidney does not start to leak glucose until a higher blood level is reached. If the body is already dehydrated, the reduction in the volume of blood makes it even harder for the kidneys to rid the body of glucose. So the blood glucose rises even higher.

As the body becomes further dehydrated, the blood pressure starts to fall and the patient gets weaker and weaker. He also becomes confused. His mental state declines until he becomes comatose.

The patient does not become very acidotic in this condition, unlike with ketoacidosis, because he has enough insulin to prevent the breakdown of fat. There is no Kussmaul breathing and no smell of acetone on the breath.

Severe infection and the failure to take insulin are other causes of hyperosmolar syndrome, but dehydration due to reduced water intake, nausea, vomiting, and diarrhea is the most frequent cause.

Symptoms

These patients have symptoms that are discovered fairly easily if anyone is paying attention to them. Among the most important are

- ✔ Frequent urination
- ✔ Thirst
- ✔ Weakness
- ✔ Leg cramps
- ✔ Sunken eyeballs and rapid pulse
- ✔ Decreased mental awareness leading to coma

The key sign of this condition is a blood glucose level of 600 or even higher.

Treatment

Hyperosmolar syndrome is a medical emergency just like ketoacidosis. The patient is taken to the Intensive Care Unit of the hospital where the emphasis is on replacing fluids and minerals that are missing, like potassium, sodium, and chloride. Surprisingly, very little insulin is required. As the minerals and fluid are replaced, the glucose rapidly falls. However, if the problem was initiated by a severe infection or injury, these issues must be treated for the patient to recover.

Dealing with Severe Long-term Complications

These problems, which occur after ten or more years of poor control of the blood glucose, are extensively discussed in Chapter 13. They include:

- ✔ Eye disease, which may lead to blindness
- ✔ Kidney disease, which may end in kidney failure
- ✔ Nerve disease, which can result in pain or weakness
- ✔ Heart disease, which usually ends in a heart attack

These complications are not inevitable. If you reverse your prediabetes so your blood glucose is normal, or if you keep your blood glucose under control when you have diabetes or prediabetes, none of these will happen.

Viewing eye disease

Diabetes may be responsible for several different kinds of eye disease. These include:

- ✔ **Cataracts:** These are opaque areas of the lens of the eye that can block your vision if they're large enough. Fortunately, a relatively simple operation can remove the cataract and replace it with an artificial lens that allows you to see normally.

- ✔ **Glaucoma:** This condition involves abnormally high pressure in the eye that can damage the *optic nerve:* the nerve through which light travels to the brain, allowing us to see. Excellent medical treatment with medications is available to lower the pressure and save the sight.

- ✔ **Diabetic retinopathy:** This condition consists of many different changes in the *retina,* the light-gathering tissue at the back of the eyeball. Some of the changes are benign, and some are dangerous to the vision, but very good treatment is available that can save your sight. Diabetic retinopathy is responsible for 15,000 to 20,000 new cases of blindness every year. But good control of the blood glucose reduces this complication by 75 percent. I discuss this complication in much more detail in Chapter 13.

Avoiding kidney disease

Your kidneys are essential for ridding your body of chemicals and toxic products of normal metabolism, as well as helping to maintain the balance of salt and water in your body. Diabetes is responsible for almost half of all new cases of kidney failure (*diabetic nephropathy*).

Diabetes affects the kidneys by damaging their filtering mechanism so they can no longer filter toxins from the blood. These poisons build up and can kill the patient if they are not removed.

One of the important ways to prevent kidney failure is to detect kidney disease in its earliest stages. Detection is done by a simple test of your urine called the *microalbumin* test. Normally, tiny amounts of protein escape from your blood and enter your urine. In the case of early kidney damage, the amount measured in the urine rises significantly above what is normally measured. In this situation, your doctor can prescribe a variety of medications to reverse the kidney damage. If the damage progresses to kidney failure, excellent treatments are still available in the form of kidney transplants and *dialysis,* a mechanical cleansing of the blood. You can find out much more in Chapter 13.

If you develop diabetes, make sure your doctor tests for microalbumin every year beginning five years after your diagnosis.

High blood glucose is not the only culprit in diabetic kidney disease. Two other abnormalities contribute: high blood pressure and high cholesterol. In treating diabetic kidney disease, you need to attack all three abnormalities. Your blood pressure should be lower than 130/80, and your cholesterol should be no higher than 200 with plenty of HDL or "good" cholesterol. Other problems, such as repeated kidney infections, can speed up the damage to the kidneys.

Detecting nerve disease

Just about any nerve in the body can be damaged by the effects of too much glucose in the blood. Careful testing may determine that as many as 70 percent of people with diabetes have nerve disease. This disease can lead to a variety of complications, which include:

- Disorders of sensation, where the person can't feel a *filament,* a hair-thin piece of plastic that is touched in several places on the bottoms of the feet. This complication may lead to amputations if an injury goes undetected and a wound forms that severely damages the limb.

- Disorders of motion, where the person becomes weak or loses the motion of certain muscle groups due to damage to the nerve that signals the muscle to move.

- Disorders of the *autonomic nerves,* the nerves that signal the heart to pump automatically or the stomach to empty automatically or the intestine to move food and wastes along automatically.

- Mixed conditions that include both loss of sensation and loss of movement.

These conditions of the nerves can make the diabetes more difficult to control. For example, if your stomach does not empty as expected, the medications that are supposed to be active as glucose is being absorbed may act too early, causing hypoglycemia. Or physical activity, an essential part of good diabetes treatment, may be curtailed by the nerve damage.

Dodging heart disease

The heart depends on blood flow from the coronary (heart) arteries to provide oxygen and nutrition to the heart muscle. If this flow is partially obstructed, the patient may experience heart pain called *angina,* especially when the heart needs to pump harder (such as during exercise). If the flow is completely obstructed, you can have a heart attack.

Coronary artery disease is the most common cause of death in patients with type 2 diabetes. In type 2 diabetes, coronary artery disease tends to be much more extensive than in people without diabetes, and even people with prediabetes have more coronary artery disease than people with normal levels of blood glucose.

If a heart attack occurs, the risk of death is much greater for the person with diabetes than for a person with healthy glucose levels. Someone with diabetes who has a heart attack has a 40 percent chance of dying from it. In contrast, someone with healthy glucose levels who has a heart attack has a 15 percent chance of dying. And after that first heart attack, the survival rate differs greatly between people with diabetes and people whose glucose is under control: Within five years after the heart attack, the mortality rate is 80 percent for the person with diabetes and 25 percent for someone with normal glucose levels.

Other factors promote coronary artery disease as well, whether or not diabetes is present. The most important are

- Obesity
- Central fat deposition (meaning you carry your fat around the waist, not around the hips)
- High blood pressure
- Abnormal blood fats, especially reduced HDL (the so-called "good" cholesterol)

Any approach to the prevention of coronary artery disease in prediabetes or diabetes must address these factors as well as the blood glucose. Chapter 13 offers much greater detail.

Facing Sexual Issues

Dick Forrest has had type 2 diabetes for 12 years. Starting around the eighth year, he began to notice that he could not maintain an erection. Reluctant at first to discuss it with anyone, including his wife, he finally brought it up on a visit to his doctor when his wife mentioned decreased satisfaction with their sex life. The doctor suggested the problem was probably associated with his diabetes. At that stage, controlling the blood glucose may have helped a little but not a lot. The doctor offered Dick some Viagra. Dick tried it and found he could maintain a firm erection for much longer, much to the satisfaction of his wife.

Jane Philburn had diabetes for 15 years with poor control of her blood glucose. Recently, she noticed that intercourse was more painful because her vagina did not lubricate the way it used to. She had frequent yeast infections, which made intimacy with her husband even less enjoyable. She saw her doctor, who suggested ways to better control her blood glucose, which seemed to take care of the yeast infections. The doctor also prescribed a moisturizing lotion that was to be administered to her vagina before intercourse. These tactics helped a great deal and restored her intimacy with her husband.

Although they are not real people, Dick and Jane could easily be patients in my practice because I see these problems every day. The sexual issues they face are typical of people with diabetes who are not in good diabetic control over many years. Up to 50 percent of males and 50 percent of females with diabetes have some disorder of sexual function.

Male sexual problems

Other factors have to be ruled out before diabetes is determined to be the culprit. Some other common causes of male sexual problems include:

- Trauma to the penis
- Medications, including blood pressure medications and medications for depression
- Hormonal disorders, such as not enough testosterone or too much *prolactin* (a brain hormone)
- Reduced blood supply to the penis due to disease in the arteries to the penis
- Psychogenic impotence, where the man has trouble only with a certain woman

I discuss treatments for male sexual dysfunction at length in Chapter 14. For now, just know that treatments are available, from pills to surgery, which can help every man.

Female sexual dysfunction

This problem is at least as common as sexual dysfunction in men, if not more so. But women seem more reluctant to discuss it than men. Or perhaps male diabetes specialists are reluctant to bring the subject up with women.

Yeast infections and dry vaginal tissues are just two of the many sources of difficulty for women with sexual problems. Other difficulties, which may or may not be due to the diabetes, include:

- ✔ Irregular menstrual function
- ✔ Feelings of unattractiveness due to the obesity that usually accompanies diabetes
- ✔ Loss of bladder control due to the nerve disease of diabetes
- ✔ A reduction in estrogen secretion in the vagina because of increasing age

Menopause can be responsible for many of these troubles, so don't assume it's the diabetes.

You can manage any of the problems mentioned here, as I explain in Chapter 14. No woman needs to suffer from poor sexual relations due to these difficulties. But you must be willing to discuss them with your physician.

Pregnancy problems

Diabetes can add a lot of burdens to the difficulties that a woman faces during the joyous occasion of pregnancy. The problems are not only the mother's, but they extend to the growing fetus. I introduce some of them here and offer more detail in Chapter 14.

Problems for the mother

Many mothers already know that they have diabetes before they become pregnant. If that's the case, it's up to them to achieve the best possible glucose control before becoming pregnant. When the baby is conceived during a period of poor glucose control in the mother, the probability of a congenital malformation (such as absence of part of the brain or splitting of the spinal column with paralysis in the baby) is much greater.

Some of the other problems that diabetes promotes in a pregnancy include:

- ✔ Difficulty in conceiving a baby in the first place
- ✔ More frequent miscarriages
- ✔ More frequent *caesarean sections* (surgery through the abdomen to remove the baby)
- ✔ The need for early delivery due to the large size of the baby

New cases of diabetes can also occur during pregnancy and are called *gestational diabetes.* This condition occurs in about 4 percent of all pregnancies. The mother does not have to worry about congenital malformations but still has to worry about the other problems listed above. She also has to worry that she will develop permanent diabetes some years after the pregnancy.

Problems for the growing fetus

Besides the concern for congenital malformations in the fetus exposed to high blood glucose during conception, there are more concerns for the fetus exposed to high blood glucose throughout the pregnancy. The fetus is able to make insulin, the storage hormone. In the presence of high glucose, more insulin is made and the fetus starts to store fat and become large in the shoulders, chest, abdomen, arms, and legs. These babies may weigh more than 8 and a half pounds (4 kilograms) at birth and create a very difficult delivery, often ending in a caesarean section.

If the father has diabetes but the mother does not, the baby is not in danger of any of these problems. The environment that the fetus is exposed to is responsible for the damage that occurs.

All the trouble that occurs for the mother as well as the growing fetus can be prevented by very tight control of the blood glucose, starting with the time before conception of the baby and continuing right through delivery.

It's vital to screen pregnant women at 24 weeks and 28 weeks of pregnancy, the time when gestational diabetes shows up. A screening test is done by feeding the mother 50 grams of glucose and measuring the blood glucose one hour after the feeding. If the glucose is less than 140 mg/dl (7.8 mmol/L), it's considered normal. If the test result is greater than 140 mg/dl, a definitive test for gestational diabetes is done, which I describe in Chapter 14.

Chapter 4

Stopping Prediabetes in Its Tracks

*I*t's time to start thinking about an overall approach to reversing prediabetes and turning yourself (specifically your body) into the person you want to be. No one can make this change for you. You have to make the decision and stick to it. Doctors can offer advice, but you meet with your doctor for just a few minutes every few months. The rest of the time you are on your own.

I'm reminded of a story told about the great saxophone player John Coltrane. He was often invited by Miles Davis, a great trumpeter, to play with his band. Coltrane had one problem. When he started playing a solo, he couldn't stop. Someone asked him why his solos were so extended, and Coltrane said, "I get involved in this thing and I don't know how to stop." Davis told him, "Try taking the saxophone out of your mouth."

The point is that you do have the power to shape your life and your health. The earlier you start, the better, because some conditions become irreversible after a time. But a good decision made even after a lifetime of bad habits can have benefits. For example, cigarette smokers are subject to sudden death. Within days of stopping smoking, your risk of sudden death greatly diminishes or even disappears. Just take that cigarette out of your mouth!

In this chapter, my goal is to get you thinking about specific actions you can take that will stop the onslaught of prediabetes and turn you back toward good health. I focus on changing your relationship with food and exercise, considering medications, and weighing the benefits and risks of weight loss surgery.

Halting and Reversing Bad Choices

Prediabetes is a consequence of a number of bad choices. Some of the most important choices include:

- ✔ The choice to eat just a little more food each day than you burn up in your daily activities, resulting in the storage of fat
- ✔ The choice to sit passively in front of a screen instead of actively moving your body for at least a half hour each day, seven days a week
- ✔ The choice to drink sugary soft drinks instead of water
- ✔ The choice to eat foods that are high in total fats, saturated fats (see Chapter 5), and trans-fatty acids and low in dietary fiber
- ✔ The choice to eat too much salt
- ✔ The choice to drink too much alcohol
- ✔ The choice to skip pills that lower your blood pressure and blood fats
- ✔ The choice not to be monitored regularly for increased glucose, increased fats, and increased blood pressure

Do you recognize yourself in this list? You may even be making additional bad choices that I didn't list here, such as using illegal drugs. Whatever bad choices you are making, they are choices. You may feel that some of them are out of your control — that you are addicted to something like food or alcohol. Even then, you have the choice to seek help. Millions of people have done so and reversed their own bad choices.

My intention is not to make you feel bad about yourself. I point out all the bad choices you are making as a way to get you to understand that you can turn those choices around into good ones. You have the power! You can take many different approaches to reversing your choices. In the sections that follow, I offer several options in the hopes that at least one will work for you.

You don't have to feel out of control. You can prevent or reverse prediabetes and avoid all the short-term and long-term complications of diabetes. You can live a long, high-quality life. You just have to start by recognizing that you have a choice.

Becoming a Brand New Shopper

Making good choices begins in the market. Chapter 15 provides an extensive approach to shopping for food. Here, I introduce you to some of the key decisions you can make to change the food shopping experience. Instead of the market influencing what you buy, you need your good instincts to determine what you carry out of the store. Follow these suggestions and you will not only improve your diet but also save money.

In doing your shopping, remember the old cliché: "Out of sight, out of mind." Here are some suggestions to maximize the healthy content of your shopping basket:

- ✔ Always have a list of what you need to buy and stick with it.
- ✔ Eat a light snack like a piece of fruit before you go to the market so you aren't hungry.
- ✔ Shop at the same market each time so you know where everything is in the store.
- ✔ Go into the market as seldom as possible.
- ✔ Don't walk every aisle. Avoid the tempting aisles like the bakery and the loose foods that often result in a little tasting.
- ✔ Get into the habit of reading food nutrition labels (which I discuss further momentarily).
- ✔ Never take a free sample. The sample items are generally high in calories and high in price. Markets want you to buy what they profit from the most.
- ✔ If you must bring your kids, give them a snack before shopping. And firmly put their high calorie, low nutrition snack choices back on the shelf.
- ✔ At the checkout lane, keep your eyes straight ahead and don't pick up the little goodies placed there to tempt you.

Focusing on fresh

One of the major new directions in eating healthy is focusing on fresh, local foods. Doing so makes great sense. Fresh foods are definitely the most delicious and nutritious way you can eat. If they come from local growers, they were picked at the peak of their taste — unlike "fresh" foods shipped from far away, which are picked before they are ripe to give them the longest shelf time. Often those foods never fully ripen, and you never get to enjoy the real taste of the fruit or vegetable. They may not even be grown for taste but only to maintain their shape and appearance before rotting.

Another major benefit of eating fresh, local food is the ability to know the farmer. Local farmers welcome direct connections to the people who buy their produce. They may put their Web site addresses on the produce so you can look up how each farmer grows his crops. Does he use sprays? Is he organic? Does he use growing methods that renew the soil?

One of the best ways to get fresh, local produce is to go to your local farmers' market. It doesn't get much better than this. You get to taste the food before you buy it — something that supermarkets are just beginning to offer. You get to talk to the farmer directly. He has often picked the crop just hours before. He can afford to let it ripen on the vine, the surest way to get terrific taste. You also get the best prices because the farmer doesn't have to pay the overhead of a supermarket or the costs of the middlemen who buy the crops and ship them to the market. Plus, many different farms are usually represented at a farmers' market. You don't have to settle for one kind of corn or broccoli. The fact that you have a choice is highly motivating to the farmer to bring the best and sell for less.

Food at farmers' markets may sometimes be a little more expensive because the farmer does not use cheap ingredients in growing it. If you can afford it, pay a little more for quality. The taste will make your investment worthwhile.

I enjoyed a five-year period when I consistently ate delicious melons, one of my favorite foods. The farmer brought them near my home hours after he had picked them. He knew how to pick a ripe, delicious melon. Even then, he insisted that I try a piece before buying the whole melon. Believe me, those melons were worth every penny I paid for them. Unfortunately, Farmer Dave and his wife got a divorce when she made him choose between her and his melons. Things were never the same.

The very best way to get fresh, local produce is to grow your own. As I write these words, a lasting recession has encouraged more and more people to garden. I have been gardening for more than 30 years. I get to choose my own varieties of tomatoes. I get to pick them when they are fully ripe and eat them minutes later. I save the cost of tomatoes in the market. I start them from seeds and show my granddaughter how a tiny seed can grow into a magnificent tomato plant. I even get to pass out tomatoes and zucchini to my neighbors because I invariably grow too much.

Try growing something yourself. If you don't have property on which to grow food, just grow some herbs on a counter in front of a window. The sense of satisfaction as you eat your own produce is worth every minute you spend growing it.

Reading labels like an expert

Packaged foods require labels to tell you what you are getting. How often do you actually read the label? It contains an enormous amount of useful information. In Chapter 15, I show you a label and go through it line by line so you know what you are reading. Here I want to point out a few of the highlights. Some of the key things to look for are

✔ **How many servings are contained in the package?** One package does not necessarily mean one serving. With some food items, that fact is obvious. (A box of pasta or rice clearly contains multiple servings.) But other times, the serving size is deceptive. (For example, some soft drink bottles that would appear to contain a single serving list their calories, sugar, and so on as if the bottle contains two or more servings.) Be warned that food manufacturers may try to trip you up in this way, and be mindful of how many calories you're actually consuming!

✔ **Is there any trans fat in the food?** *Trans fat* is a form of fat that is found in foods naturally in tiny amounts but was added by food manufacturers to increase shelf life and to replace butter because trans fat is much cheaper. It turns out that not only do trans fats raise your bad cholesterol, but they also lower your good cholesterol. Thank you, food merchants! A study in *The New England Journal of Medicine* in April 2006 showed that trans fats "increase the risk of coronary heart disease more than any other macronutrient, conferring a substantially increased risk at low levels of consumption . . . ."

Look for trans fats in margarines, cake mixes, dried soup mixes, baked goods like donuts and cookies, potato chips, candies, whipped toppings, and some "healthy" breakfast cereals. Keep trans fats completely out of your diet. The naturally occurring trans fats are okay, however.

✔ **How many calories are in a serving?** I say many times in this book that "It's the calories!" The number of calories you consume (and how that number relates to the number of calories you burn each day through exercise) determines whether you gain weight and risk moving from prediabetes to diabetes. Where the calories come from isn't the issue; how many you eat is what matters.

Your friendly nutrition label offers a lot more information as well, but I save the details for Chapter 15.

Knowing what foods and ingredients to avoid at all costs

You should avoid a few "foods" altogether. I put the word "foods" in quotation marks because these items are not nutritious but just sources of *empty calories:* calories without vitamins, minerals, or fiber. When you avoid these items, you leave room for nutritious foods that promote health. Trans fats, which I discuss in the previous section, fall into this category. The other main ones include:

- **Bleached white flour:** The bleaching process removes vitamins, minerals, and fiber, leaving empty calories. Read the food label. Look for unbleached white flour or whole wheat flour in the ingredients. Many prepared cakes and cookies contain bleached white flour. Their ingredients lists often say "enriched" white flour, suggesting that vitamins and minerals have been added back, but the result is not as good as not bleaching the flour in the first place.

- **Soft drinks with sweeteners:** A sweetened soft drink contains absolutely no nutrition. These drinks are the number-one source of energy intake in the U.S. population, but the type of energy they contain isn't what your body needs. Soft drinks contribute in a major way to the body fat that leads to prediabetes and type 2 diabetes. You should even avoid soft drinks with artificial sweeteners because they're expensive and no more thirst-quenching than ordinary tap water.

  Would you like to put me out of business? Just replace soft drinks with water in your daily routine.

- **High fructose corn syrup:** This very sweet and highly processed product contains little or no nutritional value. It's another so-called "food" that food manufacturers created. Corn starch is processed to yield glucose, which is further processed to yield fructose, a sugar that is sweeter than glucose. The fructose is then added back to corn syrup to produce high fructose corn syrup (HFCS). HFCS is about as sweet as sugar from sugar cane or beets but is much cheaper. It also extends the shelf life of processed foods. The chemicals used to make HFCS are genetically modified, so if you don't like genetic modification of your food, don't eat foods with HFCS.

Here's how to avoid HFCS:

- Limit the processed foods you eat.
- Avoid foods with added sugar.
- Don't drink soda.
- Eat fresh fruit instead of canned fruit.
- If you eat canned fruit, buy only fruit canned in its own juices.

If you go on the Internet and look for "foods to avoid at all costs," you can come up with many other suggestions, including certain artificial sweeteners, monosodium glutamate, sugar, and palm oil. But I don't yet see scientific proof that you should avoid these substances, and until I get that proof, I won't include them in this list.

Rethinking How You Eat

Changing your eating habits is tough. You learned those habits by watching your parents for perhaps 18 years. You speak like your parents, you gesture like your parents, and you probably eat like your parents, so take a good look at them. Do your parents look healthy and younger than their real age? Or do they take a lot of pills for chronic diseases that you would rather avoid?

You may have to make some big changes in your eating habits. In Chapter 16, I show you what you need to do. Following are just a few ideas to get you started.

Oh, and don't forget the wonderful new diet called the Pasta Diet! You walk past a bakery. You walk past a candy store. You walk past an ice cream shop.

Becoming your own personal chef

If you have ever built anything, you realize that one of the great pleasures is knowing where every screw, bolt, and joint is located. The same thing is true if you cook for yourself or participate in the cooking. Just as growing your own food gives you great personal satisfaction, cooking your own food makes you feel a connection to your body and your health. What are the benefits?

- ✔ You choose the ingredients.
- ✔ You choose how long to cook the food.
- ✔ You choose how much to prepare.
- ✔ You save money compared to eating out.

If you are nervous about cooking your own food, by all means take a cooking class. You can find classes for every type of ethnic food, so if you love Italian or Chinese, you can learn all you need to know to make your favorite food regularly.

Navigating a restaurant meal when you must

If you just don't feel like cooking, or if you must be away from home, you have to learn how to eat for health at a restaurant. That's a tougher assignment than you may think. You often don't know what is in the food you are eating. You always get portions that are larger than you should eat, often twice as large. Here are some things you need to know about the restaurant experience:

✔ No particular ethnic food is better than any other. You can get a healthful or an unhealthful meal in any restaurant. Some restaurants, like fast food restaurants, require more careful planning.

✔ If you choose a restaurant you can walk to and from, you get some extra exercise that helps make up for the extra calories you may consume.

✔ You can check out most restaurants' menus online and make sure they offer choices that are good for you.

✔ You can call ahead and ask if the chef will accommodate your needs. For example, ask if she will

   • Reduce the fat in a dish

   • Serve gravies and sauces on the side

   • Bake, broil, or poach rather than fry or sauté

✔ You want to find out whether the restaurant has special meals for people with diabetes. Those meals would be fine for people with prediabetes as well.

✔ You want to drink water or eat a small snack before you go so you won't be driven by hunger to make bad choices.

✔ If you reduce the calories you consume during the day prior to going to the restaurant, you allow yourself a few more calories at the restaurant.

✔ You should ask the waiter not to serve bread at your table.

✔ If you're dining with your partner, sharing one meal is ideal.

✔ You shouldn't even look at the dessert menu.

You are completely in control of the choices you make. You can get wonderful food at a restaurant and still stay within the boundaries of the plan you have made for yourself.

Getting your portions in check

When I see a new patient who is either prediabetic or diabetic, I ask the person to collect a week's worth of foods on paper. This exercise is something you can do. Don't wait until the end of the day to remember what you ate; write everything down right after eating, both the type of food and the quantity. If you wait, you may forget.

Often the food choices that the person is making are excellent. The problem is in the portions. Figure 4-1 shows the difference between the usual portions that people tell me they are eating at first and the appropriate portions of food.

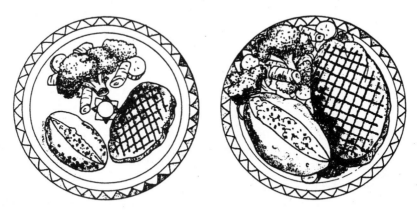

Figure 4-1: The plate on the left shows the appropriate portion size. The one on the right shows what many people eat.

You can see the difference. The larger steak has more than 600 kilocalories compared to the 220 kilocalories of the smaller steak. A modern bagel has 350 kilocalories compared to the 140 kilocalories of a bagel 20 years ago. An order of French fries now has 610 kilocalories compared to 210 kilocalories 20 years ago. Even modern coffee has sweeteners that bring a cup up to 350 kilocalories compared with 45 kilocalories 20 years ago. Is it any wonder that the population is enlarging? If you eat a mere 100 extra kilocalories daily, you gain 12 pounds in one year.

So the first advice that I have for new patients is to follow the *50 percent portion diet.* Eat the same foods that you have always eaten, but eat half as much. What a simple and amazing approach to weight loss! You don't have to give up the foods you love, just eat half as much of each.

While you're at it, take more time to enjoy your meals. Slow down the pace of your eating. You allow yourself more time to enjoy your partner and your family, and you feel full at a much lower level of food. Slowing down the pace of eating gives your brain more time to recognize that you have eaten enough.

Putting Your Body in Gear

Exercise is one of my favorite topics, and I don't just talk the talk. I walk the walk. I believe that any exercise is good for you but the most vigorous exercise is best for you. In my own case, over the age of 65, I play a hard game of squash three days a week. I use an elliptical trainer and maintain a pulse of 120 beats per minute for 30 minutes two days a week. I take walks of 5 miles a day the other two days a week to rest my body from the five hard workouts. And I lift weights, doing all the resistance exercises you find in Chapter 17 two days a week. Boy, am I exhausted! Just kidding. I have been doing this level of exercise since 1971. No one believes me when I tell them my age. The exercise makes me look and feel young, and I have never had plastic surgery.

Overcoming your fear of exercise

Are you afraid of exercise? You shouldn't be. No one says you have to wear spandex and put yourself front-and-center in an exercise class this very minute. You have lots of options close to home that allow you to get moving in a way that's comfortable to you.

What you should really fear is *not* exercising, because your body absolutely requires it. The Romans had it right: "A sound mind in a sound body." If you are older than 40 and haven't exercised in recent years, you should see your physician and get his agreement that you can exercise. He may tell you how vigorously to exercise or leave it to you to decide.

As you exercise more and more vigorously, the benefits increase dramatically. You will probably lose weight. Your mental state will improve. Other people will start telling you how well you look. And at some point you will feel a chemical high when you really exercise vigorously. That is when you are getting the most benefit, physically and psychologically. In the immortal words of the old Alka-Seltzer TV ad, "Try it! You'll like it."

Getting a walking start

In addition to having a new patient keep a food record, I ask him to buy a pedometer and keep a daily record of the number of steps he walked. After a week, I ask him to average the steps to get a daily step count. Most people are doing about 3,000 to 3,500 steps a day initially. Then I ask him to add 500 steps a day on a weekly basis. If he was averaging 3,500 steps, he should do 4,000 the next week and not move up until he has done 4,000 seven times. I get a lot of curious looks from these new patients, who can't believe they could ever get to the goal that I set for them of 10,000 steps a day. But they get there, and you can, too. In Chapter 20, I show you exactly how.

In Chapter 17, I offer all kinds of other choices for exercise as well. You don't have to jog or cycle if you don't like those activities, but you have to do something. And your exercise has to be more than just bending to your spouse's will or pushing your luck.

Adding Medications to Your Daily Routine

As of April 1, 2009, the U.S. Food and Drug Administration (FDA) had not voted to allow any medications for the treatment of prediabetes. Lifestyle change is far more efficient and successful than any medication currently available. An article in *The New England Journal of Medicine* in February 2002 reported that while lifestyle change prevented 60 percent of prediabetic people from progressing to diabetes, the best pills available could barely prevent 15 percent from progression.

Doctors can still use medications *off label,* which means the FDA neither approves nor disapproves of using the medication for that purpose. I am not suggesting that the medications I list here should be used off label, but I want to let you know what is available currently. I don't consider the use of these medications for prediabetes to be unreasonable because we know that prediabetes is associated with diabetic complications in some patients, especially eye disease and heart disease. If your doctor believes that you may benefit from medication, here are those you may hear about (which I discuss in more detail in Chapter 18):

- **Metformin** (brand name Glucophage) reduces the blood glucose by reducing the production of glucose from the liver, where it is held in a storage form called *glycogen.* Because it does not depend on stimulating insulin to work, metformin does not lower the blood glucose to hypoglycemic levels but only to normal. It has to be taken with food because it causes irritation of the stomach and intestines. Metformin is often associated with weight loss, exactly what we want in prediabetes.

- **Acarbose** (brand name Precose) works by blocking the activity of an enzyme in the intestine that breaks down complex carbohydrates like starch into simple sugars that can be absorbed into the blood stream. These complex carbohydrates are broken down lower in the intestine where the sugars can't be absorbed but cause a lot of gas, abdominal pain, and diarrhea. Acarbose does not cause hypoglycemia. I have tried it with many of my patients with diabetes, but they never like the side effects and have uniformly stopped taking it.

- **Pioglitazone** (brand name Actos) has still a different mechanism of action. It acts by increasing the sensitivity of the body to its own insulin. Pioglitazone actually reverses the primary mechanism in prediabetes and type 2 diabetes: insulin resistance. It tends to cause water retention and swelling of the legs and may worsen heart failure or promote fractures in women.

  ✔ **Exenatide** (brand name Byetta) is an injectable drug that is taken before breakfast and supper. It has some interesting actions, including causing significant weight loss in some patients. It also increases insulin sensitivity and may protect the cells of the pancreas that make insulin. These good features make me wonder why it's not always used before surgery is attempted as a treatment.

  ✔ **Sitagliptin** (brand name Januvia) is an oral agent that blocks the enzyme that breaks down the same substance in the body that exenatide is trying to emulate. That substance is called *glucagon-like-peptide 1* (GLP-1). The action of GLP-1 is prolonged. It does not have nearly the potency of exenatide, however, and I prefer to use exenatide if given the choice.

I believe these agents will be used increasingly as prediabetes and diabetes continue to explode in the population. For now they are rarely used, but you could make a good case for prescribing them earlier in someone's prediabetes treatment.

Tackling Prediabetes through Surgery

You may think that surgery should be a last resort in the management of prediabetes and the prevention of diabetes. Perhaps it should, but certainly in type 2 diabetes, no treatment has been found to be more consistently effective. In a study published in the *American Journal of Medicine* in March 2009, the authors looked at 621 studies of surgery for type 2 diabetes and found that surgery led to control or improvement of the disease in almost 90 percent of patients. The patients lost on average 64 percent of their excess body weight, and for 78 percent of them, diabetes was totally resolved. The death rate after this surgery is among the lowest of any surgical procedure.

My own opinion is that surgery should be considered much earlier in the treatment of prediabetes, especially for people considered *morbidly obese,* which means they have a body mass index greater than 40 (see Chapter 6). For a woman who is 5 feet 4 inches tall, that would mean she is about 100 pounds overweight. I might even recommend it for people with *severe obesity* — those with a BMI from 35 to 39.9 — if they have a strong family history of diabetes, other risk factors like high blood pressure and high cholesterol, and have failed more conservative treatment.

Some of the major benefits of *bariatric surgery* (surgery for obesity) are

  ✔ Significant weight loss

  ✔ Normalization of blood glucose

  ✔ Normalization of blood pressure

  ✔ Normalization of high cholesterol

✔ Improvement in heart disease

✔ Improvement in lung disease

✔ Improvement in *sleep apnea* (a condition characterized by episodes of not breathing while you're sleeping)

✔ Improvement in asthma

✔ Improvement in regurgitation of stomach contents

✔ Improvement in urinary stress incontinence

✔ Improvement in low back pain

✔ Improvement in quality of life

That's a long list. But bariatric surgery is not all positive. You must take the risks and complications into account. The decision you make must weigh the benefits against those risks and complications, which include:

✔ Death, which occurs in 1 in 300 surgeries in a good surgical center and is due to the heart disease associated with the obesity.

✔ *Pulmonary embolism* — the formation of a clot in the legs that breaks off and goes into the lungs. Sudden shortness of breath and chest pain result.

✔ Gastrointestinal tract leak from the surgery where the intestines are stapled. A severe abdominal infection can result.

✔ Bowel obstruction when scar tissue forms.

✔ Stricture where scar tissue blocks the intestine.

✔ Gallstones with pain under the right ribs.

✔ Infections such as pneumonia or abscess in the abdomen.

✔ Nutritional deficiencies like protein deficiency, vitamin deficiency, or mineral deficiency.

✔ Excessive weight loss.

None of these risks or complications of surgery (with the exception of the first one, obviously) are irreversible or permanent. And to put the risks in perspective, keep in mind that the purpose of the surgery is to prevent eventual blindness, kidney failure, nerve disease, or heart disease.

Two standard operations are now being performed for weight loss: gastric bypass and gastric banding. In each case, the word *gastric* refers to the stomach. I briefly introduce these operations here, and you can find much more detail about them in Chapter 19.

Gastric bypass

In this surgery, the stomach is divided into a small upper pouch and a large lower pouch. In addition, the small intestine is divided near where it meets the large intestine. The lower part of the small intestine is attached to the small upper stomach pouch. The large lower pouch of the stomach empties into the rest of the small intestine, which is reconnected to the lower small intestine near where it joins the large intestine. The small upper pouch of the stomach makes it impossible to eat much food at a meal, and the short length of the small intestine before it enters the large intestine significantly decreases absorption of food.

This operation results in the greatest loss of weight but also the most frequent occurrence of vitamin and mineral deficiencies. Patients who have this surgery typically lose 60 to 70 percent of their excess weight.

Gastric banding

An inflatable silicon band is strapped around the stomach, creating a small upper pouch and a large lower pouch. The small upper pouch restricts the amount of food that can be eaten, but there is no abnormal absorption of food. The band can be tightened or loosened from outside the body depending on the need for more or less weight loss. Patients who have this surgery typically lose 40 to 55 percent of their excess weight. Gastric banding has far fewer risks and complications than gastric bypass.

Part II
Food and Other Factors: Battling an Unhealthy Lifestyle

The 5th Wave   By Rich Tennant

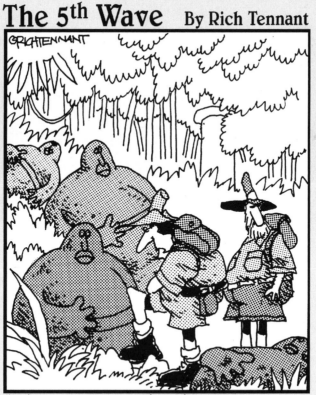

"It's a mystery why this ancient race of people died out so soon. They had an abundance of food available. The jungle here is filled with cookie bushes and the streams are full of bacon fish."

In this part . . .

The chapters in this part break down all the factors that may have led you to a diagnosis of prediabetes. First is the issue of what you have in your kitchen and why it may be contributing to your problems. Then you have to confront your weight. Being overweight is a critical factor in developing prediabetes, so I discuss the foods and forces that most often lead to weight problems. Next, I take up the important role of a sedentary lifestyle and show you how to begin to move away from it. Finally, I discuss the role of stress in your life, including how stress contributes to prediabetes and how to deal with it.

Chapter 5

What's in Your Kitchen? Identifying Problem Foods

In This Chapter

▶ Realizing how our food supply has changed

▶ Pointing out the most problematic ingredients

▶ Figuring out how eating bad foods influences prediabetes

▶ Scrutinizing your kids' eating habits

*T*ake a look in your kitchen and your pantry. There's quite a collection of food in there. Some of it is very good for you, but a lot of it should be put in the garbage, where it belongs, rather than in your body (or your child's body). How did we get to this state, where you are paying your hard-earned money for "foods" that hurt you? And I'm not talking about the constant food recalls that seem to be an everyday occurrence lately. I'm talking about a lot of ordinary food that you would do much better without.

In this chapter, I take a look at how our food supply got to the state it's in today. That food supply — along with our conversion from an active lifestyle to a sedentary lifestyle — is most responsible for promoting prediabetes and type 2 diabetes.

While we're talking about food supply, I walk into your kitchen and pantry and point out the foods that belong there and the ones that don't. I explain why the rejected foods promote prediabetes.

Finally, I look at your child's lunchbox, as well as the food offered by the school for his lunch. Is that food contributing to your child's health or encouraging eating habits that will lead to disease and early death?

These are weighty matters, but isn't this discussion exactly why you bought this book? You want to improve your health and set an example for your child. The information in this chapter can help you and your children develop healthy food habits that last a lifetime.

Understanding the Evolution of Our Food Supply

If we want to reverse our current epidemic of prediabetes and diabetes, we need to understand how we got here. And that requires knowing a little of the history of our food supply. After all, the kinds of foods that we consume tell us a lot about how we became so obese as a nation. So get ready for an extremely condensed history lesson — I promise it'll be enlightening.

Moving from forest to supermarket

We humans began as hunter-gatherers and continued to find our food in that way for thousands of years. We hunted for meat in the forest and found mushrooms there as well. We picked out the grasses that were tasty for our salads. We found wild fruits and berries on trees and bushes and ate those (not necessarily for dessert).

Believe it or not, some societies still live this way. They need to move from place to place as the food supply declines in one area and is available in another. This mobility has always tended to create a somewhat equal society because it's not possible to gather large amounts of possessions when you're constantly on the move.

The beginning of agriculture

About 10,000 years ago we started planting crops, and agriculture began. Tribes could settle in an area and store some of the crops for the months when the weather did not permit growing food. In addition, it was becoming possible to keep animals to provide more food. With settlement, it became possible to accumulate possessions, which indicated someone's status in the society and which other members of the society coveted.

Some of the new farmers were particularly adept at growing large amounts of crops, and they became the sources of food for others who were more interested in creating things with their hands. Thus began the division of labor and the trading of food for other objects. With the invention of money, it became possible to hold the value of the food or object in a convenient way until it needed to be spent on something of similar value.

The introduction of artificial fertilizers

For centuries, farmers grew crops and maintained the fertility of their lands by mixing the manure of their animals into the soil. However, at the beginning of the 20th century a scientist discovered how to turn nitrogen, a key requirement for the growth of plants, from a gas into a solid that could be spread as a fertilizer. This process allowed farms to grow crops without having animals, and it erased the limitation on the size of the farm that results from the finite amount of animal fertilizer. For the first time, farmers could set up huge farms devoted to just one or two crops.

As cities began to fill up with people who were no longer needed on the farms because of advancements in farm machinery, large markets called *supermarkets* were established to provide their food. These markets preferred to do business with as few food providers (farmers and meat raisers) as possible, leading to even more concentration.

Corn for cattle

Some people believe that the root of our current obesity problem can be traced to 1973, when a new method of supporting corn farmers was established. The government encouraged farmers to plant as much corn as they possibly could. If the price of corn fell as a result, the U.S. government would step in and pay the farmer directly. This situation led to an enormous supply of very cheap corn.

The people who raised cattle, chickens, and other animals, which had always been fed on grass, saw a way to raise more and fatter cattle, unlimited by the amount of grass available to them and using a source of very cheap calories. The animals could be concentrated in "feed lots," and their food would be brought to them instead of bringing them to the food (grass). The trouble was that cattle, especially, do not thrive when they eat a diet of corn or when they are concentrated together. They tend to get infections and have other problems that require antibiotics, so we end up eating those antibiotics. They also produce meat that is very fatty and filled with saturated fats, one of the worst kinds of fat.

Other abuses of corn

While some of the excess corn was being fed to cattle, plenty of corn was left. Food manufacturers saw this corn as an enormous source of cheap calories that they could use to produce new kinds of "food" products. They were able to put the sweetness of the corn into soft drinks, for example. While they couldn't raise the price of normal-sized soft drinks (and actually, they should have lowered the price because corn sweetener is cheaper than sugar), they began to sell supersized bottles of soft drinks.

Food manufacturers were able to extract many compounds from the corn, which they put into other foods. Here are some of those compounds:

- Corn oil
- Citric acid
- Lactic acid

- ✔ Glucose
- ✔ Fructose
- ✔ Ethanol
- ✔ Sorbitol
- ✔ Mannitol
- ✔ Xanthan gum
- ✔ Modified and unmodified starches
- ✔ Monosodium glutamate

You can find these ingredients on the labels of 10,000 to 12,000 of the 45,000 to 50,000 products found in the modern supermarket.

Through advertising and promotion, food manufacturers strongly encourage you to eat foods containing these corn byproducts. These foods are cheap to make and significantly improve the manufacturers' bottom line. But these foods may also be pushing 200 to 300 extra kilocalories into your body every day. As a result, in one year you may gain 20 to 30 pounds.

Catering to our tastes

One of our favorite flavors is sweetness. Realizing this, food manufacturers have added sweetness in the form of high fructose corn syrup to just about everything. The problems are several:

- ✔ We often don't know when to stop when we eat sweet things because our natural ability to detect that we have eaten enough calories is bypassed by sweetness.

- ✔ The foods that contain the increased sweetness are generally low in nutrition compared to foods like fruits and vegetables. Food manufacturers really don't know what is missing from the foods they make, even when they add nutrients like vitamins and minerals.

- ✔ If we try to eat healthy by choosing items advertised as "low in fat," the sweetness in those foods can undermine our intentions. The excess carbohydrates turn to fat in our bodies.

- ✔ The two largest sources of calories in the American diet, soft drinks and pastries, are made up largely of high fructose corn syrup.

Creating unrecognizable foods

Using all the components of corn, food manufacturers produce numerous products that are not actually foods but simply new combinations of those components. If you can't recognize something as food, it's not food. Just to give you an idea of what to look for so you can avoid it, here are a few examples of such products:

- ✔ **Chili's Pepper Pals Country-Fried Chicken Crispers with Ranch Dressing and Homestyle Fries:** This item contains far too much salt, saturated fat, and calories.

- ✔ **Keebler Fudge Shoppe Caramel Filled Cookies:** They're loaded with saturated fat, sugar, and calories.

- ✔ **Kraft Cheez Whiz:** You get too much fat, salt, and calories.

- ✔ **Tyson Chicken Breast Tenders:** They're filled with fat, saturated fat, salt, and calories.

- ✔ **Kashi GOLEAN Oatmeal Raisin Cookie Bar:** Sounds almost healthy, right? But it's sweetened with enormous amounts of corn-derived sweeteners and has too much fat.

Let's look at the ingredients (as provided by the manufacturer) of the last item on the list to give you the flavor of what constitutes food by the manufacturer's definition:

> Brown rice syrup *(a sweetener)*, soy protein isolate *(the protein source)*, evaporated cane juice crystals *(a sweetener)*, crystalline fructose *(a sweetener)*, Kashi seven whole grains and sesame blend, almonds, oat fiber, mechanically fractionated palm kernel oil, cocoa, rice flour, rice starch *(more carbs)*, honey *(more carbs)*, toasted soy grits, vegetable glycerin, corn grits, chicory root fiber, wheat bran, corn flour, natural flavors, salt, chocolate liquor, cocoa (with potassium carbonate), calcium carbonate, corn bran, magnesium oxide, soy lecithin, ascorbic acid, nonfat milk, vanilla extract, alpha tocopherol acetate, zinc oxide, ferrous fumerate, annatto, pyridoxine hydrochloride, folic acid, vitamin B12.

The only thing left out is the kitchen sink. Now I ask you, is this food or a chemical concoction dreamed up in a laboratory? Wouldn't an apple or an orange do the trick just as well? You know that Mother Nature has put all the ingredients for good health into those foods, and she requires no artificial coloring, flavoring, or excessive sweetness.

You could probably make a rule that anything with ten (possibly even five) or more chemical ingredients is not food. A second rule is to avoid foods that have ingredients with more than three syllables, such as *pyridoxine hydrochloride*. (Sure it's a vitamin, but you don't need it added to your food.)

Picking on Problem Ingredients

The previous section introduced you to the idea that problem ingredients abound in our food supply. Here, I want to talk specifically about some individual ingredients that you should avoid.

High fructose corn syrup

I bring up high fructose corn syrup several times in this book, with good reason. Because it's so cheap and satisfies our cravings for sweetness, food manufacturers use it in countless prepared foods. What are some of the principal problems with high fructose corn syrup?

✔ Any kind of sugar in excess is converted to fat in your liver — just what you don't want or need when you're battling prediabetes or diabetes.

✔ Fructose may actually make you feel *hungrier* as you eat more so you end up eating too many calories.

✔ Even if the sugar is not converted into fat, it's converted into glucose, which raises your blood glucose and further stresses your pancreas, possibly leading to prediabetes and diabetes.

✔ High fructose corn syrup is made from genetically modified corn, which is treated with genetically modified enzymes. If *genetic modification* is a dirty phrase in your vocabulary, avoid this ingredient.

✔ Fruit has fructose, but it also has fiber, which slows down its absorption. High fructose corn syrup lacks fiber.

Given these and other problems associated with high fructose corn syrup, do you need to eat it? The answer is a resounding no!

Refined carbohydrates

Refined carbohydrates sound like something you should add to your diet. After all, who doesn't want to be more refined, or eat things that are more refined?

But the words are meant to confuse you. As carbohydrates are *refined,* all the good nutrients are removed. Refining means that the grain has been treated with machinery to strip away the bran and the germ from the whole grain. The bran and the germ contain the vitamins and the fiber so important to your health — the ingredients that lower your risk for diabetes, obesity, heart attacks, and high blood pressure.

Why do the food manufacturers refine carbohydrates? Oils in the grain germ become rancid after a while, so refined carbohydrates have a much longer shelf life than unrefined carbohydrates. But eating them definitely doesn't prolong *your* life! Refining is not beneficial for you — only for the food companies.

An interesting study in the *American Journal of Clinical Nutrition* in May 2004 showed that the increased consumption of refined carbohydrates such as high fructose corn syrup, along with the simultaneous decrease in fiber intake, paralleled the increase of type 2 diabetes during the 20th century.

Here's how refined carbs really trip you up: You may think that a product like sugar-free cookies is better for you than a product full of sugar. But the white flour in the cookies is rapidly broken down into glucose, which is rapidly absorbed in the absence of fiber and rapidly raises your blood glucose. So I'm sorry to disappoint you, but your sugar-free bakery products are not helping!

Following is just a partial list of refined carbohydrates and the common foods that contain them — items you should avoid:

- White flour
- White rice
- Milled corn
- Candy
- Soda
- Donuts and other pastries
- Sweetened cereal
- White bread
- Granola
- White pasta

The good news is that you don't have to be hungry. You just have to make good choices. Following are some of the foods you can substitute for those in the previous list:

- Whole grains
- Beans, lentils, and peas
- Nuts and other seeds
- Vegetables
- Fruits
- Brown rice

The wrong types of fats

Fat is another word that has become almost profane. That's because we used to assume that the fat you ate would turn to fat in your body and clog your arteries. But not all fat is bad fat. Your body uses fat to make many important hormones like estrogen, testosterone, and aldosterone. It's true that fat has more calories per gram than carbohydrate or protein, but it also enhances flavor. Fat can and should be a part of your diet if you keep the fat calories under control and emphasize the right fats. The different types of fat include:

- **Saturated fat,** which is found in animal sources of fat like meat, butters, bacon, cream, and cream cheese. This fat increases levels of bad cholesterol and is much more prevalent in corn-fed cows than in grass-fed cows. Vegetable sources of more saturated (and therefore less healthy) fats are palm oil and coconut oil.

- **Trans fats,** which are naturally present in very small amounts in foods but are a huge concern because of their *unnatural* presence in our food supply. Food manufacturers produce these fats by adding hydrogen to the next group of fats, the unsaturated fats. They use trans fats to replace butter, which is more expensive. But we now know that trans fats raise bad cholesterol and lower good cholesterol.

- **Unsaturated fats,** which come from vegetable sources like olive oil and canola oil. These fats are further broken down into two groups:

  - *Monounsaturated fats* don't raise cholesterol in the blood. Olive and canola oil are in this group. Canola oil comes from a variety of the rapeseed plant that is low in erucic acid (which may be toxic) and glucosinolates (which don't taste good). The name canola comes from **Can**adian oil, **lo**w **a**cid.

  - *Polyunsaturated fats* don't raise total cholesterol but may lower good cholesterol. Examples are corn oil, mayonnaise, and some margarines.

It's not hard to realize that you want to emphasize monounsaturated sources of fat in your diet and minimize saturated fats, trans fats, and polyunsaturated fats. Fortunately, recent legislation is forcing the removal of trans fats from most foods.

Connecting Problem Foods to Prediabetes

How do problem foods encourage prediabetes and eventually diabetes? This section helps you understand why it's important to avoid them. The bottom line is that they promote obesity, which leads to prediabetes and diabetes, and they also increase the occurrence of heart disease.

Reacting to sugars and refined carbs

What happens in your body when sugars are absorbed? Why are refined carbohydrates and simple sugars so bad for you? This section gives you the complete picture of what's happening inside your body when you eat a cookie or a piece of cake.

Before table sugar (*sucrose*) enters your blood from your intestine, it's broken down into two sugars: glucose and fructose. When the glucose levels in your blood rise, the glucose passes through the *pancreas,* a small organ behind the stomach that has two major functions:

✔ To provide digestive enzymes directly into the small intestine

✔ To provide insulin directly into the blood stream

Insulin is the hormone (chemical) that opens up cells so glucose can penetrate.

When you eat simple sugars like sucrose and refined carbohydrates like white flour, they are quickly broken down and quickly absorbed into your blood stream. That's because there is little or no fiber or fat to slow down their absorption. They cause a rapid increase in the insulin levels in your blood. The result is that your cells take in glucose rapidly, and that glucose gets stored in your muscles and fat. Glucose is stored in the muscles in the form of *glycogen,* a long train of glucose molecules. In fat, glucose is stored as *triglyceride.*

If your daily intake of calories is equal to or less than your daily expenditure, you burn up all this excess glycogen and triglyceride. If your daily intake is greater than your expenditure (which is the case for anyone who is obese), you store more and more of the excess glucose. The results are fatty changes in your liver (the presence of much more fat than normal in each liver cell), weight gain, and the development of blockages in your arteries that may lead to heart attacks, strokes, or *peripheral vascular disease* (the blockage of arteries to your legs).

As you gain weight, your body's insulin becomes less effective, and you have to release more of it from your pancreas to lower the blood glucose to the same extent. This condition is called *insulin resistance.* At some point, the pancreas can't keep up. You begin to have impaired fasting glucose and/or impaired glucose tolerance (conditions I describe in Chapter 1). At that point, you have prediabetes.

Unless the impairment is reversed by weight loss and exercise, the process worsens until you reach levels of blood glucose that define diabetes. When diabetes is present, you may develop the complications that I discuss in Chapter 3. (Sometimes, complications begin even before you reach a diagnosis of diabetes.) The tendency to develop heart disease begins even in prediabetes.

The continued overstimulation of the pancreas by high glucose levels can lead to the loss of pancreatic function and even higher glucose levels.

Realizing the consequences of eating bad fat

As I point out earlier in the chapter, there are good fats and there are bad fats. Good fats like olive oil lead to improved blood flow through your arteries. Bad fats like saturated fats and trans fats can cause your arteries to become blocked.

When arteries are blocked, you may develop coronary artery disease (*coronary* means "heart"), stroke, or peripheral vascular disease (due to the blockage of arteries to your legs).

In the last three decades, the number of deaths in the United States due to heart disease has fallen dramatically thanks to all kinds of new treatments, as well as improved diets. However, the tremendous increase in the number of type 2 diabetes patients predicted for the next few decades may reverse this trend.

Remember: Stick to eating monounsaturated fats like olive oil and canola oil if possible.

Another category of fats is called *fatty acids.* They're found in fish like salmon, tuna, and halibut, as well as in nut oils and tofu. Another name for them is *polyunsaturated fatty acids.* The most important and healthful of this group are the omega-3 fatty acids. These fatty acids reduce inflammation and the risks of chronic disease like heart disease, cancer, and arthritis. Another group of fatty acids, the omega-6 fatty acids, actually promote inflammation.

The balance between omega-3 and omega-6 is important. You should consume two to four times as much omega-6 as omega-3. Most of us have no problem eating enough omega-6: Corn-fed cattle contain lots of omega-6, as do corn-fed farmed salmon. As a result, many people eat much more omega-6 than they need, and not nearly enough omega-3. This imbalance may explain the increase in inflammatory diseases in the United States. Taking omega-3 fatty acids in pill form may not provide the same protection.

Farm-raised salmon, fed on grain, may have an unhealthy ratio of omega-6 to omega-3 fatty acids. Stick to wild salmon.

Battling food addictions

Some physicians believe that harmful foods, especially sweeteners, stimulate chemicals in the brain (particularly a chemical called *dopamine*) that give an opiate-like feeling. You get "high" and want more of that feeling, so you eat more of that food.

Many doctors (including me) are skeptical that food could have the same potential for addiction as narcotics, alcohol, and sex. But how else do you explain the many people who eat large quantities of food that they know is hurting them? Doctors and others tell them to stop, but they continue to do it. Whether or not this eating behavior is based in addiction, it can be changed. Narcotics addicts, alcoholics, and sex addicts can control their behavior. And so can you if you feel that you fall into this category.

Try reducing or eliminating just one of the problem foods at a time. You'll find that you can actually live without it. If necessary, go for only a day without it and allow yourself to eat that food on the second day. Then try to skip two days, three days, and so forth. You'll be amazed at how long you can go without that food, and eventually you can give it up altogether.

When you first eliminate the offending foods, you may experience some symptoms like headaches. Try to keep at it, and the symptoms will go away.

Becoming Aware of the Glycemic Index

The glycemic index is a controversial concept in nutrition. Many doctors believe it is important and helpful, but others and certain organizations (like the American Diabetes Association) think it is too complicated for general use. I believe that the glycemic index provides important and helpful information. Even if that information is an approximation, you should understand how to use it.

The *glycemic index* (GI) is the degree to which a source of carbohydrate raises your blood glucose compared to white bread. White bread is assigned a value of 100. Another carbohydrate containing the same amount of calories is eaten, and blood glucose levels are determined and compared to the blood glucose levels found after eating white bread. Foods that raise the blood glucose half as much as white bread have a GI of 50, for example.

Studies in the *Archives of Internal Medicine* in November 2007 verify the usefulness of the GI. In one study from China, women who ate high GI rice had a significant increase in the risk of diabetes. Another study in the same journal showed a reduced risk of developing diabetes in black women who ate a diet that contained low glycemic cereal.

Select carbohydrates that have a low glycemic index if possible. You won't find refined carbohydrates in this category.

Some doctors are reluctant to use the GI more often for these reasons:

- Carbohydrates have different GIs if they're eaten alone or with other food.
- One food may have various GI counts depending on how it's processed or prepared.
- Certain low GI foods (for example, chocolate) contain a lot of fat.
- Diabetes educators are reluctant to teach about the GI because they believe it's hard to understand and creates confusion.

I believe the GI is a simple concept as long as we don't try to get too specific about numbers. We can simply suggest low glycemic substitutions for high glycemic foods and leave it at that. For example:

- Use whole grain bread rather than white bread.
- Eat unrefined whole grain cereal in place of processed breakfast cereal.
- Eat cookies made with dried fruits or whole grains instead of plain cookies.
- Eat cakes and muffins made with fruit, oats, and whole grains.
- Emphasize temperate climate fruits like apples and peaches instead of warm climate fruits like bananas.
- Eat whole wheat pasta or legumes like beans and peas rather than potatoes.
- Use basmati or other low GI rice rather than white rice.

Just because the GI is low (as in chocolate), that does not mean the food is good for you. Make sure you check the fat content before you make that food a major part of your diet.

Analyzing Your Child's Lunchbox and Lunchroom

Good eating habits must be developed at the earliest possible age. A child who is taught at home or at school that junk food and fast food are the normal diet will have a difficult time learning to eat a more healthy diet later in life.

Checking the lunchbox

What do you put in your child's lunchbox? A sandwich made of white bread, mayonnaise, and luncheon meats? Or a salad with tofu and various fruits and vegetables? After reading this chapter, you should have a pretty good idea of what to send in that lunchbox. Here are some specific suggestions:

- A green salad
- Whole grain crackers
- Fruit salad including grapes, blueberries, apples, or other seasonal fruit
- Nuts including almonds, cashews, or walnuts
- Baby carrots
- Raw green beans
- Unflavored yogurt
- A container of low-fat or nonfat milk

In other words, give him whole grains, beans, nuts and other seeds, vegetables, and fruits. Avoid processed foods with more than five ingredients that have more than three syllables in their name!

If your child has been eating healthy foods at home, you shouldn't have a hard time getting him to eat the same way at school. He already knows that he enjoys these foods, and he may even be eager to teach his friends what he knows about nutrition.

Try planting a garden, if you have the room. Send some of the produce with your child. He will be proud to show his friends that he and you grew this food, and it will be the freshest and most nutritious food he can eat.

Looking at school lunches

Unfortunately, most middle schools and high schools have vending machines that are filled with junk like soda, imitation fruit juices, candy, chips, and cookies. And if your child eats a lunch prepared in the school cafeteria, he may not do much better. School lunches often feature pizza, hot dogs, French fries, chips, cookies, and other processed and prepared foods.

The U.S. government pays for what's called the National School Lunch Program (NSLP), but the money isn't used to increase our kids' nutrition. Instead, most of the money goes for non-food items like heating the cafeteria. Foods distributed by the NSLP contain many of the same ingredients as the vending machines; they do not make up a nutritious meal.

Luckily, many parents are starting to fight back. Groups like Better School Food (`www.betterschoolfood.org`) are demanding fresh food from local farmers. Check out this group's Web site for ideas of steps you can take to make your child's lunch options healthier.

For some school nutrition success stories, go to the Web site `www.cdc.gov/ HealthyYouth/nutrition/Making-It-Happen/download.htm`. You may be inspired by what other parents have achieved in the lunchroom.

The bottom line: Don't leave your child's hot lunch choices up to the school. Find out for yourself what your child is eating in school, and improve everyone's diet by using what you have learned in this chapter to encourage good nutrition.

Chapter 6

Facing Your Weight

- -

In This Chapter

▶ Taking an honest look at your body

▶ Getting to know your BMI and body type

▶ Figuring out why you're overweight

▶ Committing to weight loss

▶ Focusing on children with weight problems

- -

*T*hink of prediabetes as a building. If you want to tear it down, you have to destroy its two foundations: excessive weight and lack of exercise. Why?

✔ When you gain excessive weight, your blood glucose goes up.

✔ When you lose excessive weight, your blood glucose goes down.

In this chapter, you and I tackle the subject of your weight. I first encourage you to get honest about the shape you're in, including finding out your body mass index number. I also highlight some of the most common reasons people in our society gain weight and offer some plain-speaking advice on how to battle temptations. I then turn my attention to a special situation: helping overweight kids so they don't turn into overweight adults.

Along the way, I show you how to calculate your ideal weight so you can figure out a weight goal. But honestly, your "ideal" weight doesn't have to be that goal. I want you to get to a weight that minimizes your health risks, particularly the risk of prediabetes and, therefore, diabetes. I'd call that weight your *healthy weight*. The number will be different for each person depending upon how much exercise you do. If you do a lot of exercise, your healthy weight will be significantly higher than if you are a couch potato. (Of course, a lot of exercise contributes to weight maintenance or weight loss, so you benefit twice!)

Looking in the Mirror, Stepping on the Scale

In my many years of medical practice (yes, I know, I should stop practicing and start doing it for real already!), I have met a number of people who refuse to know their weight. Getting weighed is one of the first things a patient does in my office, so staying ignorant of that number can be pretty tough. But these people close their eyes when they get on the scale, or they turn around so they're weighed backward and don't have to see the reading. They ask my assistant not to tell them. When they come into my office, they ask me not to tell them even before they say hello.

Facing facts

Sometimes ignorance may be bliss, but these people are not happy. They know they're too heavy. They know they have gained weight. I don't understand how they benefit by not knowing their precise weight. Do they believe that if they don't know the number, it can't be true? If they don't acknowledge the severity of the problem, will it go away?

If you look up *ignorance* in the dictionary, the word is defined as "uneducated, unaware, uninformed." These characteristics don't always lead to bliss, but they can certainly lead to trouble, especially when the ignorance relates to your health. Preventative medicine is based on the premise that you find out you have a medical condition in its earliest stages and do something about it while the condition is still minor.

I believe a more useful maxim is "knowledge is power." You can begin to manage a problem only if you accept that the problem exists.

I recently had a former patient in my office who is clearly overweight. She was expressing concern about her daughter, who is only 10 years old and already quite heavy. She told me that her daughter is not slim like her. Clearly, this person doesn't acknowledge her own condition. As a result, she very likely won't do a thing about it.

Sizing up your status

The first step in managing your overweight condition is to make measurements. Here's what I suggest:

✔ Take a digital photograph of yourself and print it out so you have a "before" image you can look at.

✔ Buy yourself an accurate scale and use it to take an accurate measurement of your weight. Write that weight on the back of the photograph.

✔ Calculate your body mass index (BMI) using the information you find in the next section. Write your BMI on the back of the photograph as well.

✔ Measure the size of your waist with a tape measure. While you're at it, measure your arms, hips, and legs at some spot of your choosing. Write all that information on the back of the photo.

✔ As you lose weight, take a photograph and make the same measurements at least once a month. Doing so creates a record of your success, your setbacks, and your ultimate journey to excellent health. And if, in the future, you find yourself needing to lose weight again, this record will remind you that success is possible.

Becoming Familiar with Your Body Mass Index

Here's a riddle for you: How can a 125–pound person be underweight, normal weight, overweight, and obese? The answer: One person cannot be all these things at the same time. But four different people who weigh exactly the same can fall into these four different categories:

✔ A man who is 5'8" tall and weighs 125 pounds is underweight.

✔ A woman who is 5'3" tall and weighs 125 pounds is normal in weight.

✔ Someone who is 4'10" tall and weighs 125 pounds is overweight.

✔ A person who is 4'6" tall and weighs 125 pounds is obese.

Obviously, height is the factor that determines whether or not a person is normal weight. Your body mass index (BMI) looks at both your weight and height to determine whether or not you are normal weight.

If you are good with math or have a calculator handy, you can figure out your own body mass index. You just need to know your weight in pounds and your height in inches. Here's what you do:

1. Multiply your weight in pounds by 703.

2. Divide that result by your height in inches.

3. Divide that result by your height in inches again.

For example, say you are 5'4" tall and weigh 125 pounds. Multiplying 125 by 703 equals 87,875. Dividing 87,875 by 64 (inches) equals 1,373. Dividing 1,373 by 64 equals 21. What does the result mean?

- ✔ A body mass index of 18.5 to 24.9 is normal.
- ✔ A body mass index of 25 to 29.9 is overweight.
- ✔ A body mass index of 30 and above is obese.

So at a BMI of 21, you would be considered to have a normal weight for your height.

To make your life easier, Table 6-1 does your BMI calculation for you! Find your height in inches in the left-hand column. Move along that row to the right until you reach your weight. Your BMI is at the top of that column. Each BMI is expressed in kilograms per meter squared.

If you find it easier to track your BMI over time using an online tool, tag this Web site as a favorite: www.nhlbisupport.com/bmi. This service of the National Heart, Lung and Blood Institute lets you plug in your height in feet and inches and your weight in pounds and click once to get your BMI.

Want still another option? A less complicated (but also less accurate) assessment of the appropriate weight for your height uses one formula for men and another for women:

- ✔ **Men:** You should weigh 106 pounds if you're 5 feet tall. Add 6 pounds for every inch above 5 feet. For example, at 5'5", you should weigh 136 pounds (106 pounds plus 30 pounds for the additional 5 inches). Because no two people have the exact same ideal weight, you calculate your ideal *range,* which is plus or minus 10 percent from that central number. Our 5'5" fella could weigh as much as 14 pounds less or 14 pounds more than 136. So the normal range for a 5'5" male would be 122 to 150 pounds.
- ✔ **Women:** You should weigh 100 pounds for 5 feet, plus 5 pounds for every inch over 5 feet. So a 5'4" woman should weigh 120 pounds: 100 pounds plus 20 pounds for the 4 inches. Plus or minus 10 percent means 12 pounds below or above that number, giving a range of 108 to 132 pounds.

While it's important to know your ideal weight, from my perspective you need to aim for your *healthy* weight. Several studies have shown that you can be a little heavy and still be healthy, so don't stress too much if you're slightly above the high end of your ideal weight range. Just make sure you're getting plenty of exercise.

Table 6-1   **Body Mass Index Chart**

Body Mass Index (kg/m²)	19	20	21	22	23	24	25	26	27	28	29	30	35	40
Height (Inches))	Weight (Pounds)													
58	91	96	100	105	110	115	119	124	129	134	138	143	167	191
59	94	99	104	109	114	119	124	128	133	138	143	148	173	198
60	97	102	107	112	118	123	128	133	138	143	148	153	179	204
61	100	106	111	116	122	127	132	137	143	148	153	158	185	211
62	104	109	115	120	126	131	136	142	147	153	158	164	191	218
63	107	113	118	124	130	135	141	146	152	158	163	169	197	225
64	110	116	122	128	134	140	145	151	157	163	169	174	204	232
65	114	120	126	132	138	144	150	156	162	168	174	180	210	240
66	118	124	130	136	142	148	155	161	167	173	179	186	216	247
67	121	127	134	140	146	153	159	166	172	178	185	191	223	255
68	125	131	138	144	151	158	164	171	177	184	190	197	230	262
69	128	135	142	149	155	162	169	176	182	189	196	203	236	270
70	132	139	146	153	160	167	174	181	188	195	202	207	243	278
71	136	143	150	157	165	172	179	186	193	200	208	215	250	286
72	140	147	154	162	169	177	184	191	199	206	213	221	258	294
73	144	151	159	166	174	182	189	197	204	212	219	227	265	302
74	148	155	163	171	179	186	194	202	210	218	225	233	272	311
75	152	160	168	176	184	192	200	208	216	224	232	240	279	319
76	156	164	172	180	189	197	205	213	221	230	238	246	287	328

Identifying Where You Carry Your Fat

In recent years, physicians have learned to make a distinction between subcutaneous fat and visceral fat:

- *Subcutaneous fat* is located between your skin and the wall of your abdomen, arms, legs, and chest.
- *Visceral fat* is deeper in the abdomen, surrounding the abdominal organs.

Although subcutaneous fat is more visible, visceral fat is more dangerous to your health. Visceral fat produces belly fat (the "beer belly" or "pot belly").

Finding the danger in visceral fat

Whether or not you like it, as you get older, the amount of fat in your body slowly increases. For women, around the time of menopause, as levels of the female hormone estrogen fall, the distribution of fat shifts from your arms, legs, and hips to your abdomen. The less you exercise and the more you eat, the greater your tendency to form visceral fat. Visceral fat is associated with one or more of the following health risks:

- Prediabetes
- Diabetes
- Heart disease
- Metabolic syndrome
- Breast cancer
- High blood pressure
- Gallbladder disease
- Cancer of the colon and rectum

Why is visceral fat more dangerous? This type of fat is not just sitting around waiting to be used for energy. It produces hormones such as estrogens. This fact may explain the increased tendency to develop breast cancer, especially after menopause. Visceral fat also produces other hormones that increase insulin resistance, leading to the metabolic syndrome (see Chapter 9) and diabetes.

How much visceral fat can you gain before you increase your risk of disease? Dr. Abel Romero-Corral and others at the Mayo Clinic have shown that a "Modest Gain in Visceral Fat Causes Dysfunction of Blood Vessel Lining in

Lean Healthy Humans: Shedding Weight Restores Vessel Health." This study was presented at the American Heart Association's Scientific Sessions in November 2007. The researchers looked at two groups of volunteers who had normal body mass indexes. One group was assigned to gain weight (only 9 pounds), while the other group's members maintained their normal weight. The results were extremely interesting:

- The weight gainers increased their visceral and subcutaneous fat significantly.
- Blood flow in the weight maintainers remained normal and unchanged.
- Blood flow in the weight gainers decreased.
- After the excess weight was lost, normal blood flow was restored.
- Visceral (not subcutaneous) fat levels correlated with the decrease in blood flow.

Here's what the study says to me: Even small gains in visceral fat in normal weight people lead to abnormal changes that may predispose someone to a heart attack or a stroke.

Measuring your waist

The easiest way to determine if you have too much visceral fat is to measure your waist line. If you are a woman and your waistline is greater than 35 inches, you have too much visceral fat. If you are a man and your waistline is greater than 40 inches, you have too much visceral fat.

If you're Asian, this broad rule won't work for you. Studies have shown that Asians can have increased visceral fat even when their waist circumference is normal. And they tend to develop the risks of disease at a lower weight than Caucasians. The dangerous waistline size for Asian men is considered to be 35 inches. For Asian women, the number is 31.5 inches.

To do a proper measurement of your waistline, run a tape measure around your bare body at the level of the top of the hip bone. Measure your waist circumference after breathing out normally, and don't pull the tape measure so tight that it indents your skin. Don't suck in your stomach. You may get a lower reading that way, but it won't be accurate.

You can tell a lot about visceral fat by looking in the mirror. If you have the shape of an apple, which is larger in the middle, you have a tendency to develop visceral fat. If you have the shape of a pear, which is larger at the bottom, your fat is more subcutaneous.

The good news is that after you begin to diet, the first fat that goes is the visceral fat. A loss of just 5 to 10 percent of your body weight can significantly reduce the risks associated with visceral fat. Even more good news is that exercise, especially vigorous exercise (such as a brisk walk for 30 minutes a day, six times a week), can prevent the accumulation of visceral fat. A study published in *The Journal of Applied Physiology* in October 2005 showed that vigorous exercise reduced visceral as well as subcutaneous fat even with no change in food intake.

Realizing How You Got Here

If you're overweight, you probably have spent many years getting to your current condition. In this section, I explore some of the routes you may have taken during those years. Understanding each one can provide you with the opportunity to change to a healthier lifestyle. Adding up all the changes can get you back to a body that promotes good health rather than the health risks I discuss in the previous section. Remember: When you feel great, that's when you can hit a home run!

Eating out

Eating out is a real challenge, especially if you indulge in the *killer B*: the buffet. The buffet is the reason you can lose your shirt in Las Vegas but you can't lose weight there. My first advice is to avoid restaurants that feature buffets. The temptation to fill your plate multiple times is just too great. After all, weren't you told by your dear mother that it's a crime to leave food on your plate?

Noting the problems you run into

Numerous issues make eating out difficult. Here are a few:

- You have no idea what's in the food, and studies show that we generally underestimate the calories in restaurant food.
- The meal may be delayed, and you may end up eating and drinking in the bar before the meal.
- Restaurant portions are almost always too large.
- Many easy-to-order foods take hours to prepare so people order them in restaurants instead of making them at home.
- The descriptions of the foods on the menu, especially the desserts, make them hard to resist.
- Hamburgers, French fries, and pizza are the top three U.S. favorites for eating out.

The Food and Drug Administration published a report in 2006 that the restaurant industry didn't appreciate. The report suggested that the excess calories being eaten by Americans are coming from restaurants.

Preparing to go to a restaurant

You can do several things before you get to the restaurant to decrease your chances of overeating:

✔ Look at the menu on the Internet and make choices before you get to the restaurant. You are much more likely to make good choices this way.

✔ Feel free to choose any type of ethnic food, but avoid buffets.

✔ Consider a local restaurant so you can walk to it and burn some calories on the way.

✔ Find out if the restaurant has special meals for people who want to control their calories.

✔ Drink water or have a vegetable snack before you go, to lessen your appetite.

✔ Call and find out if the restaurant will allow you to substitute lower calorie choices (like a vegetable) for higher calorie choices (like French fries). For example, the restaurant may

- Provide skim milk instead of whole milk

- Reduce the amount of butter, sugar, and salt in a dish

- Serve dressings and gravies on the side

- Bake, broil, and poach rather than fry or sauté

Keeping your control at the restaurant

After you arrive at the restaurant, take these steps to reduce your risk of eating too much:

✔ Don't arrive early. If you do, you may sit in the bar and order a drink (and snack on the salty items found there).

✔ Tell the host you need to be seated promptly.

✔ Keep bread off the table if possible.

✔ Ask for raw vegetables as you wait for the food.

✔ Plan to take half your food home.

✔ Order wine by the glass and have only one.

✔ Remind yourself that soup and salad can make a delicious low-calorie meal.

✔ Keep in mind that a vegetarian dish may not necessarily be good for you. It may contain a lot of fat. Check it out by asking the waiter.

Miscalculating portions

Restaurant rule #1: The portions of food on your plate are always more than you should eat, often by a factor of two. If you eat half of what they serve you, you are probably eating the right amount. I call that "Dr. Rubin's half-portion diet." You can eat the other half at home the next night, and the meal will actually cost half as much!

Why are restaurant portions so large? Restaurants supply what diners demand. When I was writing *Diabetes Cookbook For Dummies,* 2nd Edition (Wiley), I asked the same question of many of the chefs who provided recipes for the book. They all said the same thing: Americans want a lot of food on their plates — much more food than European diners want, for example.

And because we're so used to seeing heaping portions of food when we dine out, our ideas about portion sizes get skewed even when we're preparing our own food at home. After all, if the restaurant offers a half-pound burger, why would you make anything smaller when you're grilling in your backyard?

But, of course, we *should* make something smaller at home. No one needs to consume 8 ounces of beef at one sitting, or four slices of bread, or a heaping pile of potatoes . . . We simply don't need so much food on our plates.

So what *do* you need on your plate at mealtime? Let me start by making some comparisons between ideal food portions and other objects that you can easily visualize:

- ✔ Three ounces of meat, fish, or poultry is the size of a pack of cards.
- ✔ A medium fruit is the size of a tennis ball.
- ✔ A medium potato is the size of a computer mouse.
- ✔ An ounce of cheese is the size of a domino.
- ✔ A cup of fruit is the size of a baseball.
- ✔ A cup of broccoli is the size of a light bulb.

A pack of cards, a light bulb, and a baseball should make a delicious low-calorie lunch.

Misreading your appetite

One common reason that people eat too many calories is they misread their appetite. Your appetite is a very subjective feeling. The definition of appetite is the desire to eat food, felt as hunger. The purpose of your appetite is to regulate your energy intake. If you already have large amounts of stored energy, you shouldn't have an appetite. Yet most often, you still do.

For example, consider a 5'4" female who weighs 160 pounds. Her ideal weight is 120 pounds, so she has 40 pounds of stored energy. Each pound contains about 3,500 kilocalories of energy, so this lady is carrying around 3,500 x 40 or 140,000 kilocalories of stored energy. One minute of walking uses 4 kilo-calories, which means that she could walk for 35,000 minutes (24 full 24-hour days) before she would use up her stored energy, assuming she ate nothing during that time. Chances are she would feel hungry *long* before she used up all those stored calories. Her hunger, however, would not be due to lack of energy, but to habit.

"What do I do if I'm hungry?" my overweight patients often ask me. I ask in return, "What happens if you ignore the hunger?" The answer is invariably, "Nothing."

Most hunger is habit, especially if you are overweight. If you simply ignore the sensation of hunger, you'll likely not experience any bad consequences.

Craving the wrong kinds of foods

If we would just crave carrots and celery, none of us would have any weight problems. Unfortunately, we usually crave stuff like doughnuts and choco-late. And if you give in to the craving and indulge in the doughnut or choco-late, your blood glucose rises. Then your body's insulin rises in response, sometimes sending your blood glucose too low, creating hunger. To appease the hunger, you eat more doughnuts or chocolate, of course.

We can break food cravings into two types:

- **Psychological cravings:** These cravings reflect what you want, not what you need. They spur emotional eating.

- **Physiological cravings:** These cravings reflect what you need. Your body is actually low on energy and has no stored supplies of carbohydrates or fats.

Most craving is psychological. When you eat sweets, your body releases a chemical called *serotonin* in your brain, which makes you feel happy. That's why certain sweets like chocolate have come to be associated with positive emotions like love.

You can overcome these cravings for the wrong kinds of food. Here are a few tips:

- ✔ Eat more protein.
- ✔ Eat high fiber foods, including whole grains.
- ✔ Don't eat refined foods such as white rice, white flour, or refined sugar.
- ✔ Eat small, frequent meals (such as every three hours).
- ✔ Wait for the craving to go away without feeding it.
- ✔ Get plenty of exercise.
- ✔ Don't skip meals.
- ✔ Get enough sleep.
- ✔ Occasionally allow yourself a little of what you crave.

Knowing That You Can Lose Weight

In the previous section, I offer a slew of tips to get you started on the path toward weight loss. In Part V of this book, I give you lots more ideas of how to shop, cook, eat, and exercise your way to a healthy weight.

I want to emphasize that little things mean a lot. A small weight loss of 5 to 10 percent of your current body weight can significantly reduce your health risks. That means if you weigh 200 pounds, a loss of 10 pounds will make a big difference, and 20 pounds will make a huge difference. You may go from blood glucose levels that define prediabetes to levels that are normal just by making that much progress with your weight.

Additionally, just a few minutes a day of very intense exercise or 30 minutes a day of less vigorous exercise can bring you back from prediabetes to normal. I talk much more about exercise in the next chapter and in Chapter 17.

Put together a little weight loss with a little exercise, and you can amaze your friends and startle your relatives.

Here are a few other things you can do to encourage weight loss:

- ✔ **Get enough sleep:** Lack of sleep increases your appetite. Aim for eight hours a night. After all, while you're sleeping, you can't be eating!
- ✔ **Avoid foods with pesticides:** Pesticides change hormones in a way that results in more fat.

✔ **Keep antidepressant use to a minimum:** These medications often cause weight gain.

✔ **Marry a thin person:** Two heavy people almost inevitably produce heavy children.

✔ **Reverse your usual thinking:** Think of vegetables as the main ingredient of your meal and meat, fish, or poultry as the side dish.

Helping an Overweight Child

Between 1980 and 2006, the prevalence of obesity in children between 6 and 11 years of age more than doubled from 6.5 percent to 17 percent. Almost one of every five children in the United States is obese. I said *obese,* not just overweight. Children generally do not grow out of obesity; they have to be helped out. Without intervention, there is a 70 percent chance that an obese child will become an obese adult.

When I see a very overweight child in my office, I'm saddened to know that the child could be suffering from the complications of diabetes (like blindness and kidney failure) at a very young age, just 10 to 15 years after a diagnosis of diabetes is made.

Obesity has extreme effects on children. In addition to prediabetes and diabetes, obese children suffer from bone and joint problems, stopped breathing during sleep (*sleep apnea*), high blood pressure, and social and psychological problems. They are often shunned by other children and have low self-esteem.

If you are the parent of an obese child, you can do a lot to help:

✔ **Set an example!** Your child looks to you for the right way to eat and how much exercise to do. Plus, improving your own eating and exercise habits will benefit you as much as your child.

✔ **Make movement a priority:** Encourage your child to go out for sports in school, and make sure the school has a program of exercise. More than 60 percent of high school students do not meet recommended levels of physical activity.

✔ **Know what your child is eating:** As I discuss in Chapter 5, make sure you know what your child is getting from his or her school lunchroom. If the selections aren't healthy, be vocal about the need for improvements, and insist that your child carry a lunch to school in the meantime.

Chapter 7

Stuck on the Couch:
The Risks of Being Sedentary

*I*f you don't exercise, you are missing out on the single most important, simplest, and least expensive tool for good health and long life that exists. Exercise can have a profound effect on prediabetes, diabetes, and the chance that prediabetes will proceed to diabetes. These are key long-term reasons to exercise. In the short term, exercise, especially vigorous exercise, promotes the secretion of pleasure hormones in your brain. As one of my friends who exercises regularly and vigorously says when I ask him how he is feeling, when you exercise you "couldn't be better."

In this chapter, I explain the function of exercise both for your body and for your brain. I discuss how depression affects your willingness to exercise (or do anything else, for that matter) and how to fight against that inertia. I reveal how you likely got into the habit of not exercising and what you need to do to get out of it and make exercise a part of your daily life.

How can I convince you to exercise? On a comedy album featuring the character "The 2,000 Year Old Man," Carl Reiner asks Mel Brooks, "What was the means of locomotion 2,000 years ago?" Brooks says, "What d'ya mean, locomotion?" Reiner asks, "What was it that got you to move quickly from one place to another?" Brooks answers, "Fear."

I hope to make knowledge, not fear, the reason you start to "move quickly from one place to another."

Understanding the Essential Role of Exercise

Exercise has numerous benefits. Here is just a short list of some of them:

- ✔ Exercise prevents prediabetes from becoming diabetes.

- ✔ Exercise prevents *macrovascular disease:* the disease of any of the large blood vessels in the body. In other words, it prevents heart attacks, strokes, and *peripheral vascular disease* (the blockage of arteries that serve the legs).

- ✔ Exercise increases your self-esteem.

- ✔ Exercise reduces your risk of osteoporosis.

- ✔ Exercise reduces your risk of breast cancer.

- ✔ Exercise increases your strength and stamina.

- ✔ Exercise reduces depression (see the next section).

- ✔ Exercise diminishes the effect of stress (which I discuss in Chapter 8).

- ✔ Exercise can help you maintain weight loss or even cause weight loss if it's done for a sufficient amount of time.

- ✔ Exercise lowers your blood pressure.

- ✔ Exercise tones and firms your muscles.

- ✔ Exercise may help you to overcome substance abuse like cigarette smoking and alcoholism.

Remember, you don't get the benefits of exercise by shopping faster, eating more briskly, and pushing your luck. And while it's true that exercise kills germs, it's not easy to get them to exercise.

In the following sections, I look at a few of these benefits in some detail.

Stopping prediabetes from becoming diabetes

Numerous studies have shown that insulin action, fasting blood glucose levels, and glucose intolerance are all improved by exercise. One of the most important studies was published in *BMC Endocrine Disorders* in January 2009. Sixteen men aged 19 to 23 did just 7½ minutes of very high intensity exercise on a stationary bike per week for two weeks. That small amount of exercise led to a very significant improvement in their insulin sensitivity.

If you are over 35 years old and have not exercised much before, you must visit your doctor for a consultation before you begin highly vigorous exercise.

Is it unrealistic for you to consider high intensity exercise? I don't think so. Start with 10-second "spurts" of activity with 30-second rests in between. Gradually build up to 30 seconds of high intensity with 30 seconds of rest between. Do that sequence five times in a row, and you are exercising at the same level as the people in the study.

A second important study (reported in *Applied Physiology, Nutrition, and Metabolism* in June 2007) looked at the scientific evidence for the effect of exercise and concluded that "30 minutes per day of moderate- or high-level physical activity is an effective and safe way to prevent type 2 diabetes in all populations."

So whether you want to go all out and get your exercise over with in 7½ minutes a week, or whether you want to work at a lower intensity and do 30 minutes a day, you can delay and perhaps prevent developing diabetes by exercising.

Preventing heart attacks, strokes, and peripheral vascular disease

The evidence that exercise can prevent macrovascular disease such as heart attacks, strokes, and peripheral vascular disease is just as strong. An article in the *Mayo Clinic Proceedings* in April 2009 made two important points on this subject:

✔ Physical activity, exercise training, and overall cardiorespiratory fitness can prevent these diseases — the evidence is overwhelming.

✔ For someone who already has cardiovascular disease, exercise can prevent it from recurring. (Unfortunately, patients don't use cardiovascular rehabilitation programs nearly often enough.)

Besides lowering your blood glucose, exercise prevents macrovascular disease by creating the following effects:

✔ It lowers your blood pressure.

✔ It lowers your total and bad cholesterol while raising your good cholesterol.

✔ It lowers your stress levels.

These effects occur in all age groups, including the elderly and children. Bottom line: You are never too young or too old to exercise and benefit from it.

Increasing your self-esteem

From kids to adults, daily exercise reduces symptoms of depression and improves self-esteem. How do we know? In one study at the Medical College of Georgia, kids aged 7 to 11 exercised for either 20 or 40 minutes each day after school for 13 weeks. Both groups of kids experienced improved self-esteem, but the 40-minute group benefited more than the 20-minute group. The kids did aerobic exercises like running, jumping rope, and playing basketball and soccer.

Many studies show that older people experience the same esteem benefits from exercise. For example, a study from the Department of Psychology at Bishop's University asked 127 men and women to fill out questionnaires that assessed their self-esteem, body satisfaction, and body build. With both genders, people who exercised a lot reported higher self-esteem than people who didn't exercise much.

It doesn't seem to matter what kind of exercise you do. Increased self-esteem is a side effect whether you play a sport, do martial arts, do weight training, or run.

Reducing your risk of osteoporosis

Osteoporosis is a loss of bone tissue that occurs with age in both sexes and is exacerbated by the loss of the hormone estrogen when women hit menopause. If you lose too much bone, you can suffer from fractures in your hips and spine. Your doctor can determine your level of bone loss by doing a *bone densitometry study:* The lower the densitometry, the more bone you've lost.

Weight-bearing exercises seem to be best for preventing osteoporosis. *Weight-bearing* means that you exercise on your feet, with your bones supporting your weight. Dancing, using an elliptical training machine (which is easy on your joints), climbing stairs, gardening, and walking are examples of weight-bearing exercises. Swimming is not because the water, rather than your bones, is bearing your weight. Bike-riding is also not a weight-bearing exercise because you are sitting.

Other types of exercise, like resistance exercise and flexibility exercise, are also necessary. When you do *resistance* exercise, you use your bones and muscles against the weight of some other object. *Flexibility* exercises improve your balance and prevent injuries. Some examples that you can choose from include:

✔ Regular stretching

✔ Tai Chi

✔ Yoga

I show you some specific resistance exercises and offer some advice about stretching in Chapter 17.

Maintaining or increasing your weight loss

If you've already lost weight, you can maintain that loss with exercise. But it takes a bit more exercise to actually lose more weight. The key in both situations is to do some moderate-intensity exercise for a long enough time.

The best information concerning how much exercise you need to maintain weight loss can be found in the National Weight Control Registry (www. nwcr.ws/). Begun in 1994, it has been following thousands of people who have maintained at least a 30-pound weight loss for one year or longer. Members have lost an average of 66 pounds and kept the weight off for 5.5 years. Here are just a few stats gleaned from this registry:

✔ Loss of weight has been as low as 30 pounds and as high as 300 pounds.

✔ "Losers" have kept it off from 1 year to 66 years.

✔ "Losers" have lost weight rapidly or taken as long as 14 years to lose their weight.

✔ Walking is the most frequent form of physical activity for the registry members.

✔ Most members follow a low-fat, reduced-calorie diet.

✔ 90 percent of members exercise, on average, one hour per day.

What if you want to lose more pounds? The American College of Sports Medicine recommends at least 250 minutes of moderately vigorous exercise a week to lose weight. With that much exercise and just a small reduction in daily kilocalories (say 200 kilocalories), you can lose about a pound a week. In three months, you will lose 12 pounds. Even without reducing your food intake at all, you may lose 2 pounds in three weeks.

Examples of moderate-intensity exercise are

✔ Walking 2 miles in 30 minutes

✔ Playing doubles tennis

✔ Dancing rapidly

✔ Jogging 1 mile in 14 minutes

✔ Swimming slowly

The dynamics of exercise

Exercise increases your body's demand for both glucose and fat for energy. The glucose leaves your liver and the fat leaves your fat tissue, and they both go to your muscles. Here's how these processes happen when you exercise:

✔ The storage form of glucose in the liver (called *glycogen*) breaks down and releases its glucose. After the glycogen is used up by continued exercise, your liver can make large amounts of glucose from *amino acids,* the building blocks of protein.

✔ If you exercise at a steady and moderate pace, your glucose production decreases and your body turns to fat for energy.

✔ If you exercise very vigorously, your liver produces more glucose. Sometimes the glucose production outpaces the use of the glucose by your muscles, and your blood glucose rises for a while. Vigorous exercise usually doesn't last very long, and the extra glucose replenishes your muscles when the exercise ends.

Bottom line: Glucose is your energy source when you exercise vigorously, and fat is your energy source during less intense exercise. To lose fat, focus on steady, moderate exercise.

You don't have to put in as much time if you do vigorous exercise. You need to find out for yourself how much time is necessary for weight loss, depending on how vigorously you exercise. Examples of vigorous exercise are

✔ Jogging 1 mile in 12 minutes

✔ Playing singles tennis, squash, or racquetball

✔ Running 10-minute miles

✔ Dancing vigorously

✔ Skiing downhill or cross country

✔ Rowing, canoeing, or kayaking vigorously

✔ Bicycling at 10 to 16 miles per hour

Using Exercise to Combat Depression

People get depressed for many reasons. Sometimes the depression is an appropriate response, such as when you lose a loved one, a home, or a job. But sometimes you feel depressed and don't understand why.

For someone with a health condition such as prediabetes, depression is especially problematic because you simply can't take optimal care of yourself when you're depressed. You're much more likely to make poor food choices, overeat, and exacerbate your health problems when you're struggling with depression.

Medications and psychotherapy may help, but exercise should be part of any plan to combat depression. In this section, I explain why.

Inactivity contributes to depression

Confession time: Doctors don't know everything. (I'll pause while you recover from your shock.) One thing we don't know is exactly how lack of exercise contributes to depression. However, we have some theories, including these:

- ✔ Exercise raises the level of *neurotransmitters* in your brain: the chemicals that permit your brainwaves to move. This increase tends to improve your mood. Without activity, these chemicals are not secreted.

- ✔ Exercise raises your levels of *endorphins:* chemicals that are like physiological opium. Endorphins help you to sleep better, decrease tension in your muscles, and decrease the production of stress hormones like cortisol in your body.

- ✔ Exercise raises your body temperature slightly, which may have a calming effect.

Lower levels of neurotransmitters and endorphins may lead to anger, anxiety, fatigue, sadness, and many other symptoms associated with depression.

Depression contributes to inactivity

When you are depressed for any reason, you tend to lose interest in yourself and your environment. You develop an "I don't care" kind of attitude. Under these circumstances, you are not interested in being careful about what you eat, taking your medications, and doing exercise.

This situation qualifies as a Catch-22: a no-win situation. (The concept comes from the novel *Catch-22* by Joseph Heller. One of the novel's characters is an airman who is crazy and should not be allowed to fly missions during World War II. But if he asks to be grounded, that action would be considered sane, and therefore he'd be allowed to fly.) You're depressed and don't want to exercise. And because you don't exercise, your depression doesn't improve.

If you don't find a way to break out of this no-win situation, you'll likely continue to struggle with depression. For specific ideas of how to break the cycle, read the "Planning to Move" section at the end of this chapter.

Unraveling the Typical Excuses

Lots of factors (including depression) lead to a lack of exercise. Over the years, I've probably heard just about every explanation (or excuse) from my patients. In this section, I highlight some of the biggies and explain why none of them have a leg to stand on.

Lacking time

Many excuses come down to this reason. People are so busy with other things that they can't find the time to exercise. Many patients tell me that their children monopolize their time or they work long hours, for example.

This excuse rings hollow for two reasons:

- No one is completely efficient in their use of time. In other words, if you study your daily schedule and get real about where your time is actually spent, you *will* find that you can carve time out to exercise each day. Don't believe me? Read the "Finding time" section later in the chapter.

- The time you spend exercising will pay off by improving your health and lengthening your life. In the short run, you'll have more energy, which will improve the quality of time you spend with family, at work, and so on. In the long run, you'll be around longer in order to spend time doing all those things you love!

Loving your TV or computer

This factor goes hand-in-hand with the whole issue of lacking time to exercise. Simply put, we spend huge amounts of time daily in front of the television and the computer.

The Council for Research Excellence studied the behavior of 350 adults in ten-second intervals over three years. It found that adults are exposed to one screen or another (TVs, mobile phones, movies, GPS devices, monitors) for 8½ hours a day. We spend, on average, a little over *five hours* in front of the TV each day.

Do you really need to look at a screen for a full one-third of your day? No wonder you have no time to do anything else!

Think your life would be miserable without your TV or computer time? Researchers at the University at Buffalo, The State University of New York were curious what would happen if children were denied access to TV and computer screens. They followed 70 children ages 4 to 7 for two years. All the kids were in the heaviest quarter of their age group. Half were allowed to watch TV as usual while the other half watched only 50 percent of their usual time. The researchers used a device called the TV Allowance attached to the TV to control the amount of TV viewing. Here's what the study discovered:

- Television viewing is directly related to the consumption of fast foods and other foods and beverages advertised on TV.

- Viewing cartoons with embedded food commercials increased preschoolers' desire for the advertised items.

- After two years, 30 percent of the children who decreased their TV time went from overweight to normal weight. Only 18 percent of the control group made that kind of progress.

- The amount of exercise remained the same for both groups. The difference was that kids who watched less TV decreased their daily food intake by 100 kilocalories.

The American Academy of Pediatrics recommends no more than two hours of TV or computer time daily for children 2 and older and none for younger children.

What's true for children is true for adults A study by the Healthy Active Living and Obesity Research Institute at the Children's Hospital of Eastern Ontario showed that adults who watched more than 21 hours of TV a week were 80 percent more likely to be obese than people who watched 5 hours or less. Here are some possible explanations for this finding:

- Watching commercials and watching TV characters who eat and drink prompt us to eat and drink more.

- TV viewing can lead to mindless, repetitive eating. You can pretty quickly consume a whole bowl of chips without thinking.

- You make poor food choices in front of the TV. When was the last time you ate carrot sticks while watching your favorite show?

- Watching TV burns only slightly more energy than sleeping.

Plus, all this TV time may prevent you from spending time preparing healthy meals. You're more likely to eat unhealthy prepackaged meals or takeout instead. Too much TV viewing can also create stress because you're wasting time and not doing tasks you need to accomplish.

Convincing yourself that exercise is too hard

This roadblock to doing enough exercise usually results from trying to do too much too soon. If *A* is no exercise and *Z* is exercise that makes a real difference in your health, you can't go straight from A to Z. You must pass B, C, D, and so on. If you try to do too much too quickly, your body rebels. The aches and pains build up, and you shut down.

A simple and obvious solution is to build up very gradually. Doing so is much better for your health than undertaking too much strenuous exercise all at once.

Consider an example: You want to become a jogger but have not jogged before and are not in particularly good shape. After you check with your doctor, you can proceed in the following way:

- ✔ Day 1: Jog for 15 seconds.
- ✔ Day 2: Jog for 30 seconds.
- ✔ Day 3: Jog for 45 seconds.
- ✔ Day 4: Jog for 60 seconds.

And so on. You need a stopwatch or a good watch with a second hand. The best device is one you can set to alarm you when the right amount of time has passed.

Using this method, in just four months, you'll be jogging 30 minutes a day, and it will seem effortless. Don't jump the gun! By the time you reach 10 minutes or so, you may be tempted to tack on more than 15 seconds each day. But what's the hurry? By adding just 15 seconds a day, you assure yourself that you can do it and avoid injuries that set you back. In fact, if you need to, you can stay at any given level as long as you want (or need) before moving up.

After you've reached the 30-minute mark, you have two choices:

- ✔ Continue to lengthen your workout by 15 seconds daily until you get to 45 minutes or more.
- ✔ Intensify your workout by trying to go a little faster so you cover more distance in the same 30 minutes.

You can follow the same procedure for resistance training (weight lifting). Start with just 2.5 pounds of weights. In this case, the next level may be 5 pounds, so instead of moving up every day, stay at each level for a week. If the next level is too difficult, go back to the previous level until it becomes easy, and then move up. Figuring out how much weight you eventually want to lift is a little tricky. I discuss this subject a lot more in Chapter 17.

Yes, exercise is too hard if you try to do too much too soon. But if you approach it in a gradual manner, it becomes something that you not only *can* do but *want* to do. You'll welcome the challenge to prove to yourself and others that you can do it.

Planning to Move

So what steps do you have to take go from a couch potato to a buff tomato? Here are some suggestions:

- ✔ **Start with a realistic goal:** For example, in four months I want to be able to jog for 30 minutes. Or in three months I want to be able to lift 60 pounds over my head 18 times.

- ✔ **Break the goal down into small improvements:** For example, each day I want to add 15 seconds to the duration of my jogging. Each week I want to add 5 pounds to the weights that I lift over my head.

- ✔ **Gather the equipment you need:** It may include a set of weights, a stopwatch, or even a GPS training watch. This wonderful device, made by many manufacturers (including Garmin, Timex, and others) allows you to

  - Measure the time of exercise

  - Measure the distance of exercise

  - Measure the speed of exercise and change it "on the run"

  You can alter your workout easily by adding time, adding distance, going faster, or combining any of those changes.

- ✔ **Consider starting with a personal trainer:** These highly trained individuals can make sure that you are doing your exercise properly from the beginning. You're much better off learning the right way to exercise at first — otherwise, you have to unlearn the wrong way. Explain to your trainer that you are not in a hurry; you want to build up gradually, but you have a definite goal.

In case any of the obstacles (or excuses) that I discuss in the previous sections are still holding you back from a commitment to exercise, let me address them one by one.

Exercising through your depression

I want you to try an experiment. Make yourself laugh even if you don't have anything to laugh about. Just perform the physical act of laughing. As you continue to laugh, I can almost guarantee that you'll begin to feel happier. You are performing the end result of amusement, and you start to feel amused. This is essentially what happens when you listen to a good comedian. He starts you laughing (presumably by saying something really funny), and after a while, everything is funny.

You can accomplish the same thing with exercise and depression. Start walking for just a few seconds a day. The feeling that you can actually do something will begin to alter your perception that you can't do anything. Your perception will change even more if you continue to add seconds and prolong your exercise each day. You may still need a psychologist and medications to help you, but you also may find that as you do more and more exercise, you can leave those other tools behind.

Finding time

The best way to overcome this roadblock to exercise is to examine how you spend your time each day. For one day, write down what you do every minute, starting the moment you wake up. For example, here's how I spent my day yesterday:

- ✔ 6:15: Awoke
- ✔ 6:15-6:20: Bathroom
- ✔ 6:20-7:00: Looked at e-mails and *The New York Times* online
- ✔ 7:00-8:24: Wrote part of *Prediabetes For Dummies*
- ✔ 8:24-9:15: Breakfast
- ✔ 9:15-9:20: Bathroom
- ✔ 9:20-12:30: Wrote part of *Prediabetes For Dummies*
- ✔ 12:30-1:15: Lunch
- ✔ 1:15-5:00: Wrote *Prediabetes For Dummies* plus bathroom
- ✔ 5:00-5:30: Exercised on the elliptical trainer
- ✔ 5:30-6:15: Showered, shaved, and dressed

✔ 6:15-7:15: Supper

✔ 7:15-9:05: Watched a movie

✔ 9:05-10:30: Read e-mails, wrote *Prediabetes For Dummies,* bathroom

✔ 10:30-6:18: Sleep

I managed to get in my 30 minutes of exercise, but I could have done more. Most of the e-mails were junk mails, and I could have just deleted them. I could have skipped reading *The New York Times* online — most of the news was gloom and doom anyway. I could have spent a little less time writing this book. I could have shortened my meals by just a few minutes, although meal times are restful for me and an opportunity to spend quality time with my wife. I could have skipped the movie, although I love movies and this was a good one. The point is that I probably *could* have found two hours or more in the day to do more exercise, if doing so were a priority.

Try doing the same time study for yourself. You may be amazed by how much time you can find to do a little more exercise. I've always found it curious that the busiest people I know seem to have the most time to do what they need to do.

What if your time study reveals that the only way to exercise is to sleep even less than you already do? If you simply can't do 30 minutes of exercise each day, start by making time to do 2½ minutes of high intensity exercise every day. Just that small amount can make a huge difference in your health, both physically and mentally.

Turning off your TV or computer

You need to set screen-time boundaries, not just for your children but for yourself. Outside of your work hours, limit yourself to a maximum of two hours of screen time a day (including TV, computer monitors, cell phones, and GPS devices).

If you can't accomplish this goal on your own, get a device I mention earlier in the chapter: the TV Allowance (www.tvallowance.com). Set it for yourself, as well as for your kids. And don't forget that your kids tend to do as you do, not as you say. Use your newly found extra time to demonstrate to your kids the importance of exercising, reading, preparing healthy meals, and so on.

You *do* have enough time, enough energy, and enough motivation to exercise. You don't have to strive to become a world-class athlete — just to do enough exercise to prevent going from prediabetes to diabetes and to move back from prediabetes to a healthy state.

Chapter 8

Stressing Out

*Y*ou can't avoid stress. You likely experience it in your job, in your family, in your relationships, in the world around you, and within yourself. And stress can make you sick if it causes you to stop eating properly, maintaining your hygiene, taking necessary medications, protecting yourself against contagious disease, and exercising.

In this chapter, I point out possible sources of stress in your life — both those you can change and those you can't. I discuss how stress affects your food intake and may contribute to prediabetes. I offer suggestions for minimizing the impact of stress in your life. And finally, I discuss the special situations of stress for the elderly and for kids.

Just remember, if you look hard enough, you can always find a silver lining — even in the face of terrible stress. Think about the man who went to his doctor and told him, "I look in the mirror and think I'm looking at a dead man. My face is thin, my cheeks are hollow, my skin is sallow, my hair is falling out. What is it?" The doctor said, "I don't know, but your eyesight is perfect."

Recognizing Sources of Stress in Your Life

Feelings of stress are normal. Your body responds to various threats (both physical and psychological) with a fight-or-flight reaction. The result is the production of hormones such as adrenalin and cortisol, both of which raise your blood glucose to provide more fuel for your muscles and brain. These hormones have side effects, which make you aware that you are under stress. What are some of the side effects?

- Your hearts pounds.

- Your chest muscles contract, and you have trouble breathing.

- You *hyperventilate,* which means you breathe too rapidly and feel light-headed.

- Your arms and legs become shaky.

- Your throat feels tense.

- You clench your jaw.

When you're under stress, you may develop one or more symptoms, which are divided into four major categories: physical, emotional, behavioral, and cognitive. Here are some of the biggies:

- Physical symptoms

  - Aches and pains

  - Diarrhea or constipation

  - Frequent colds

  - Loss of sex drive

- Emotional symptoms

  - Depression

  - Feeling overwhelmed

  - Irritability

  - Moodiness

- Behavioral symptoms

  - Isolating yourself

  - Eating too much or too little

  - Developing nervous habits, like nail biting

  - Neglecting responsibilities

✔ Cognitive (thinking) symptoms

- Anxious thoughts

- Constant worrying

- Inability to concentrate

- Poor judgment

You can see what a profound effect stress can have on your health. I say more about that connection later in this chapter.

Categories of stress

You should be aware of different kinds of stress:

✔ *Acute stress* results from a recent situation or problem or a problem you anticipate in the near future. For example, an auto accident, a deadline for a report, or a robbery can cause acute stress. Because the stressors are short-term, this type of stress isn't as damaging as other kinds. You may have symptoms such as a pounding heart, dizziness, or headaches, but they subside as the acute stress subsides.

✔ *Episodic acute stress* occurs in people who live very disorganized lives. These people are overburdened with responsibilities that they can't manage. They are highly competitive, hostile, and insecure, and they have constant headaches, chest pain, and gastrointestinal symptoms like diarrhea. Treating episodic acute stress is much more difficult than treating acute stress because the disorganized lifestyle is so ingrained in the individual. People in this situation often need long-term professional help.

✔ *Chronic stress* results from situations that go on and on, such as the situation in the Middle East between Arabs and Jews or a long-term unhappy marriage. People with chronic stress feel trapped and may give up trying to solve the problem. Often they go on living their lives hopelessly and die of a heart attack or suicide. These people are the most difficult to treat because they feel certain that they are "stuck."

Stressors can be further divided into those you can change and those that are out of your control. Some of the stressors may seem like happy events to you (like an engagement, a new baby, a new house, or a new job), but they are still sources of stress.

Stressors you can change

You may like to believe that you have control over just about everything (except death and taxes), but some situations are easier to change than others. Please don't misunderstand me: When I say "easier," I don't mean "easy." In truth, the process of changing any source of stress in your life often causes additional stress! Your task is to determine if the increase in short-term stress will result in a decrease in stress in the long haul. For example,

- ✔ If you're engaged but not certain that the marriage will be right for you, you may be better off breaking the engagement.

- ✔ If you're in a very stressful marriage, divorce (despite the stress it creates) may ultimately be your best choice.

- ✔ If you have ongoing problems with a friend, a neighbor, or a relative, you may need to take action that is difficult in the short term but will pay off by reducing your stress later.

- ✔ If you're in a financial mess, you likely need to make some tough choices now (such as taking a second job or cutting out any unessential expenses) that will reduce your long-term stress.

- ✔ If you've got legal problems, you're probably better off facing any tough consequences now rather than trying to delay them. The stress will only increase with each day that your situation remains in limbo.

Stressors out of your control

Many stressors fall into this category because they're created by other people or events that you can't control. Some common examples of stress outside your control include:

- ✔ Buying or selling a home (because of a work relocation, for example)

- ✔ Separating from a loved one

- ✔ Getting a divorce (if your spouse is the one instigating it)

- ✔ Losing your job and starting a new one

- ✔ Retiring (even if you've been looking forward to it)

- ✔ Getting emotionally or physically ill

- ✔ Watching a spouse, family member, or friend go through a bad illness

- ✔ Experiencing the death of a spouse, family member, or friend

- ✔ Getting pregnant and giving birth

For a much more extensive list of stressors, check out `http://stresscourse.tripod.com/id14.html`. At this site, you can find a checklist called "Cooper's Life Stress Inventory." You check off the stressors in your life and select the severity of the stress from 1 (low level) to 10 (very severe). You add up the numbers and grade yourself. If you score 100 or more, you are under high stress.

Assessing Your Attitude toward Your Stressors

How you perform under stress is greatly affected by your personality. Each of us has a set of personality traits, many of which are similar to other people's traits. These sets of traits categorize us as *Type A* or *Type B* personalities. Many people have traits that fall in both sets, but most of us have traits that predominate in one group or the other. Table 8-1 shows how Type A and Type B personalities differ.

Table 8-1	Type A and Type B Personality Traits
Type A Traits	*Type B Traits*
Always in a hurry	Never in a hurry
Can't quietly listen	Listens until the other person is finished
Doesn't like to wait	Waits calmly
Excessively competitive	Not excessively competitive
Holds feelings in	Can express feelings
Must finish things	Can leave things unfinished
Never late	Unhurried about appointments
Minimal social activities	Many social activities
Tries to do several things	Does one thing at a time
Wants everything perfect	Can accept imperfection

Looking carefully at yourself

As you look at Table 8-1, you may find it relatively easy to see where you fit in. The traits on the left are tight and tense. If you see yourself on that side of the table, you are subject to high stress. Events in your life trigger stress reactions that are not good for your health. You are subject to the signs and symptoms of stress that I list earlier in the chapter. You may also be depressed, feel overwhelmed, overeat, or worry constantly.

If you identify more with the right side of the table, you are probably pretty laid back. When stressors come along, you take a more philosophical attitude. You think more in terms of "This too shall pass." You are much less likely to be made sick by stress than someone with a Type A personality.

Of course, many people are in denial. They can't see themselves clearly. You may want to ask others (especially a spouse) to provide some input about which side of the table you fit in. But generally speaking, if you feel constantly under pressure, you're very likely a Type A personality.

Giving yourself a break

If you're a Type A personality, you may be setting yourself up for sickness. When you react with a fight-or-flight response, you are using an ancient coping behavior that's often not useful for modern sources of stress. Sure, if the stress is a car that is about to hit you, the flight response is exactly what you need. Those types of circumstances are rare, however. Most of the stressors I list in this chapter require you to think calmly about the problem and solve it if possible.

The way we think about the stress plays a major role in our ability to handle it. Back in 1917, Italian playwright Luigi Pirandello (who won the Nobel Prize for Literature in 1934) had the first performance of his play *It Is So (If You Think So)*. He went on to write a number of plays with the same theme, which is this:

> The way we think things are determines our reaction to them, whether our observation of things is true or not!

Pirandello wasn't the first person to write on this theme. It goes back to the ancient Greeks, but Pirandello's plays made it explicit. Characters in his plays are constantly misinterpreting what they observe and damaging themselves or others by their reactions.

Take the example of losing a job. For one person it may be a highly stressful event that provokes worries about finances and the ability to take care of his family, undermines his self-esteem, and so forth. For another the same event may represent a chance to stop doing something that he found uninteresting or tedious or something that didn't pay enough. He may have the perspective that he now has an opportunity to take a break and rethink his career.

The take-home message is that how you think about a situation determines whether you respond with a smile or with sickness.

What personality traits are most helpful in meeting the stresses that come our way? Dr. Susan Kobasa studied executives at the Bell Telephone Company while it was being restructured in the late 1970s and observed that three important personality traits were present in executives who did not respond to the stress with sickness. They were:

- **Commitment:** Committed people are involved in their families, their work, and their communities. This commitment motivates them to work harder and gives them a purpose.

- **Control:** People have one of two traits when it comes to control:

    - An *internal locus of control,* which means you believe you have some influence on external events

    - An *external locus of control,* which means you think you are simply an observer in life, and everything that happens to you is due to destiny

    Obviously, people with an internal locus of control believe that they can do something about a stressor, which is healthier than the alternative.

- **Challenge:** This term refers to the way you see the stressor. Do you see it as something to be overcome or as something that will overcome you? People who can deal with a challenge accept that change is inevitable. They welcome change as a chance to learn something new.

Winifred Gallagher is the author of a book called *Rapt,* which is about the science of paying attention. A 2009 article about her in *The New York Times* explains that several years ago, she was being treated for a severe form of cancer. She said, "When I woke up in the morning, I'd ask myself: Do you want to lie here paying attention to the very good chance you'll die and leave your children motherless, or do you want to get up and wash your face and pay attention to your work and your family and friends? Hell or heaven — it's your choice."

These three traits — commitment, control, and challenge — are not necessarily built in to your DNA. They are *learned,* and everyone — including you — can learn or unlearn them. So give yourself a break, and learn how to cope with stress without getting sick.

Linking Your Stress Level to Your Relationship with Food

People under stress tend to consume foods that aren't good for their health. They eat fast foods, drink a lot of caffeine, eat foods that are high in fats and refined carbohydrates, and drink alcohol. A study by the American Psychological Association in 2006 indicated that 41 percent of women use food to deal with stress. People are especially susceptible during the holiday season, when lack of time, lack of money, and the pressure to give gifts are major stressors. In Chapter 5, I discuss the negative effects of eating that kind of diet over a long period of time.

Studies at the University of California in San Francisco have shown that one normal response to the secretion of stress hormones (especially cortisol) is to search for pleasurable food such as chocolate, pastries, and other sweets. These foods are called "comfort foods" for a good reason.

Another study in the *Family and Consumer Sciences Research Journal* in January 2008 looked at the "Effects of Stress on Eating Practices Among Adults." Two-thirds of 185 university faculty said they changed their eating habits when stressed: 70 percent increased their food intake, and 30 percent decreased their food intake. When stressed, they chose more sweets and salty/crunchy foods.

The logical explanation for all these research results is that sweet foods give us the glucose that we need for the fight-or-flight response. However, other things are going on. One is that most of us are taught as children that we get a treat in response to sadness or physical discomfort. (Maybe your mother would give you a cookie after she cleaned off your scraped knee.) In addition, when we're stressed, we pay less attention to what we're putting in our mouths. Stress also causes us to drink a little extra alcohol to dampen the pain.

Finally, stress — particularly chronic stress — causes a number of symptoms and even diseases that result in problems with food. It forces an alteration in diet that may not be helpful to the person with prediabetes. Among the medical symptoms and diseases that stress can provoke are

- Colitis: An inflammatory disease of the large intestine
- Gastritis: Inflammation of the stomach
- Irritable bowel syndrome: Cramping, abdominal pain, bloating, constipation, or diarrhea that does not permanently harm the intestine

✔ Obesity

✔ Stomach and duodenal ulcers

✔ Stomach pain

Avoiding Exercise Because of Stress

Just as we tend to eat too much of the wrong kinds of foods in a stressful situation, we also tend to stop exercising. A 2006 survey by the American Psychological Association showed that people under stress tend to discontinue their exercise program. They turn to sedentary behaviors like watching TV, sleeping, overeating, and drinking to manage their stress, especially during the holidays.

Stopping exercise is exactly the wrong reaction to stress because exercise is such an important part of reducing stress. I discuss your body's need for exercise (especially during stressful times) in depth in Chapter 7.

Realizing How Stress Contributes to Prediabetes

By now, you should have a pretty clear sense of how stress contributes to prediabetes. Stress causes us to do many of the things that predispose us to prediabetes and to stop doing things that prevent it. In response to stress, we tend to

✔ Stop exercising

✔ Stop eating carefully

✔ Use poor judgment

✔ Avoid contact with people who could help us

✔ Believe that we have no control over our lives and stop trying

When all these negative behaviors are taking place, the chances of you developing prediabetes (and diabetes) increase significantly.

Understanding Stress in the Elderly

The elderly are subject to sources of stress that are different from children and younger adults. Here are some of the most frequent sources of stress in the elderly:

- Declining health
- Decreased strength, mental ability, and balance
- Reduced income
- The sickness or death of a spouse
- The sickness or death of other relatives and friends
- Fear of an attack at home
- Social isolation (as friends and relatives die)

All these stressors, and many others, can easily lead to end results such as poor eating habits, lack of exercise, and other physical behaviors that are extremely detrimental. That's one reason that this age group has the largest number of people with prediabetes and diabetes.

If you recognize yourself (or a loved one) in the description I'm offering here, you can take a number of steps to reduce the stresses that seem inevitable for the elderly:

- **Get involved in group activities:** Socializing with other people the same age can help you learn about solutions that others have discovered. If nothing else, it gives you the opportunity to vent to people who understand what you're experiencing.

- **Take time to relax and rest your body:** At the same time, don't stop doing exercise because it can help so much to reduce stress.

- **Be extremely careful about what and how much you eat:** Your metabolism is likely slower than it used to be, which means you may gain weight easily.

- **Avoid cigarettes and alcohol**

- **Get enough sleep**

- **Learn something new:** Start to do something you've always wanted to do but never had enough time for, like playing the piano or speaking a new language.

In a study published in *Adultspan Journal* in March 2009, elderly people living in nursing homes were questioned about how they cope with stress. They mentioned the following three methods most often:

✔ Praying

✔ Reading, watching TV, or listening to music

✔ Talking to friends and family

While there's nothing wrong with any of these methods, focusing on healthy food and exercise need to be high on the list of coping mechanisms as well.

Perceiving Stress in Kids

Unfortunately, young people aren't immune to stress. Even though they don't have to pay bills or hold down jobs, kids have their own stressors that are as significant for them as adult stressors are for you. The following sections describe common stresses for kids and how to reduce them.

Identifying sources of stress

Kids have plenty of stresses. The stresses can be external (like the expectations of parents) or internal (like their desire to fit in socially). Some of their major stressors include:

✔ Separation from parents when they have to go to preschool or school

✔ Pressures of school and social activities

✔ Pressure from having to keep up with too many activities, including schoolwork, athletics, and music lessons

✔ Sympathetic stress from hearing the troubles of their parents

✔ Sympathetic stress from learning about world problems (like poverty or disease)

✔ Divorce or other family problems

Reducing stress

Kids need the help of adults to reduce their stress because they may not see a way out on their own. Here are some of the things you can do to help them:

- **Listen:** Offer a sympathetic ear. Sometimes just being heard is enough to reduce stress substantially.

- **Reduce the schedule:** If your child is overscheduled, suggest eliminating some activities.

- **Be honest:** Don't try to sugarcoat or minimize divorce, financial problems, or other family issues. Chances are your child already knows how severe the problem is, so discuss it openly with him or her.

- **Offer perspective:** Put world problems into perspective for your child. For example, the world economy may be bad, but your own family is doing fine.

- **Reduce screen time:** Free up time for homework, outside activities, and exercise by getting your kids away from the TV and computer.

- **Think like a child:** Anticipate and prepare your kids for things that they find stressful, like dentist's appointments.

Part III
Getting a Diagnosis

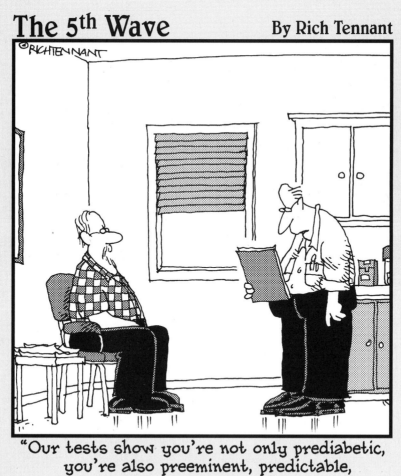

The 5th Wave   By Rich Tennant

"Our tests show you're not only prediabetic,
you're also preeminent, predictable,
and precocious."

In this part . . .

Prediabetes is associated with another abnormality that is called the *metabolic syndrome.* You find out about this syndrome here. You also discover the kinds of tests that you and your doctor should do so that you have a complete picture of your metabolism. When it comes to securing a diagnosis, children and the elderly have some special considerations, which I present in this part as well.

Chapter 9

Spotting the Metabolic Syndrome

*I*f you've read some or all of the chapters that have come before this one, you know that I talk a lot about the necessity of a healthy lifestyle. So far, my focus has been solely on getting healthy in order to prevent or reverse prediabetes. In this chapter, I turn your attention to another condition that develops as a result of an unhealthy lifestyle: the metabolic syndrome. The metabolic syndrome goes by many other names: *metabolic syndrome X, syndrome X, insulin resistance syndrome,* and *CHAOS.*

Why am I bringing up this condition in a book about prediabetes? Two reasons:

✔ The two conditions have a great deal in common. Their causes are similar, and the threats they pose to your body are equally severe.

✔ You combat the metabolic syndrome just as you do prediabetes: by changing your eating habits, getting more exercise, and taking other steps to improve your lifestyle.

So if you're concerned about prediabetes, chances are you need to be concerned about the metabolic syndrome as well. And if you're willing to take the necessary steps to halt and reverse prediabetes, you'll get twice the bang for your buck because you'll be combating the metabolic syndrome at the same time.

In this chapter, I explain exactly what the metabolic syndrome is, how to determine if you're at risk, what lab tests are done to achieve a diagnosis, and what steps to take to get back to good health. Not bad for just 12 pages!

Defining the Metabolic Syndrome

Like prediabetes, the metabolic syndrome is a condition that is often associated with *visceral* obesity, which means obesity that involves carrying your extra weight around your waistline (as opposed to in your hips and thighs, for example). If you have an apple-shaped body type, chances are you've got too much visceral fat.

However, just to keep life interesting, you don't have to be overweight to be diagnosed with the metabolic syndrome. If you have other risk factors and develop the signs and symptoms of the condition (which I describe in this chapter), you need to see your doctor even if you're thin.

As early as 1947, patients who showed signs of the metabolic syndrome were described by a French physician. This doctor made the connection between upper body obesity and diabetes, coronary heart disease, high cholesterol, and gout.

But only in 1988 did Dr. Gerald Reaven propose (in a lecture to the American Diabetes Association) that insulin resistance is the underlying cause of the metabolic syndrome. As I explain in Chapter 2, *insulin resistance* occurs when the insulin in your body stops working effectively.

The metabolic syndrome shares a lot of the features of prediabetes and responds to similar treatment. Having the metabolic syndrome can also predispose you to developing diabetes. Current estimates indicate that up to 25 percent of the U.S. population has the metabolic syndrome. Left untreated, this condition can lead to a fate similar to that of diabetes: a fatal heart attack.

New research suggests that the metabolic syndrome may also be associated with higher rates of cancer and worse outcomes for cancers of the breast, prostate, large intestine, and other organs. Excess insulin may stimulate the growth of tumors.

Determining Your Level of Risk

In this section, I explain who is most at risk for the metabolic syndrome. Having a single risk factor is not something to panic about. However, if you recognize yourself in several of the descriptions that follow, you definitely want to schedule a chat with your doctor about this condition.

Having a genetic predisposition

Most studies of the metabolic syndrome indicate that there is a hereditary component. Here are two key reasons for this conclusion:

- ✔ The metabolic syndrome tends to cluster in families.

- ✔ When *identical twins* (twins from a single egg) are compared with *non-identical twins* (twins from two different eggs) for the development of the features of the metabolic syndrome, the identical twins have common features of the metabolic syndrome much more often.

However, identical twins do not *always* match up for the development of the metabolic syndrome. In other words, one twin in the set may develop the metabolic syndrome, and the other may not. This fact suggests that lifestyle and environment also play a part in developing the condition.

Getting older

As people get older, the incidence of the metabolic syndrome increases greatly. Only 9.2 percent of women between the ages of 20 and 29 have the metabolic syndrome. In contrast, 64.4 percent of women between the ages of 80 and 89 have it. For men, the percentages are 11.0 percent in the younger group and 47.2 percent in the older age group.

Unfortunately, you can't do anything about aging (just as you can't do anything about your genetic heritage). Fortunately, you *can* take action in response to the remaining risk factors. Keep reading to find out how.

Gaining weight

As you gain *visceral* fat (the kind that accumulates around your belly), your body's insulin becomes less effective. Your pancreas has to pump out more insulin to get energy into your muscles. This loss of insulin effectiveness is called *insulin resistance.* As you push more glucose into your cells, you are also creating more fat, and you gain more weight. The result is a further increase in insulin resistance. At some point your insulin can no longer keep up, and your blood glucose rises into the diabetic range.

Here's the kicker: You may develop the metabolic syndrome even if your weight is completely normal! One study showed that men with a body mass index (BMI) of 25–26.9 were more than twice as likely to have the metabolic syndrome as men with a BMI of 18.5–20.9, but the latter group *did* have cases of the metabolic syndrome. (I explain BMI in Chapter 6.) So even if you're thin, you're not immune to this condition.

Slim people who have the metabolic syndrome are said to be *metabolically obese*. The phrase implies that even though their weight is in the normal range, their metabolism is similar to that of an overweight person.

If your BMI is toward the high end of normal, and if you recognize that you have signs and symptoms of the metabolic syndrome (which I describe in the next section), you need to lower your weight further. I provide a BMI chart in Chapter 6 so you can see exactly where you stand.

If you are obese, the metabolic syndrome may be one more reason to consider bariatric surgery (see Chapter 19). When patients with the metabolic syndrome undergo bariatric surgery, up to 75 percent of them lose the signs and symptoms for the metabolic syndrome as they lose weight.

Living a sedentary lifestyle

Another major factor in developing the metabolic syndrome is living an unhealthy lifestyle. If you don't get much physical activity and you consume excess calories, you are living a lifestyle that promotes the metabolic syndrome. The sedentary lifestyle is strongly associated with the signs and symptoms of the metabolic syndrome.

Here's the great news: You can take control of this risk factor. When people with the metabolic syndrome follow an exercise program for 20 weeks, up to 30 percent of them no longer have signs or symptoms of the metabolic syndrome!

How insulin resistance develops

As visceral fat accumulates, it acts differently than *subcutaneous* fat (fat that is located between your skin and the wall of your abdomen, arms, legs, and chest). Insulin usually causes fat storage, but visceral fat resists that action and releases large amounts of substances called *free fatty acids*. These excessive free fatty acids in the blood cause resistance to insulin in the liver and muscles, with these results:

✔ The production of new glucose is stimulated in the liver.

✔ The muscles take in a reduced amount of glucose from the blood.

As fat cells become filled, they resist the storage of additional fat, and it starts to be stored in your muscles, liver, and pancreas, further increasing insulin resistance in those organs.

Another substance produced by visceral fat is an enzyme that causes the production of more cortisol. *Cortisol* is a hormone that increases the distribution of fat in the waist area and causes even more insulin resistance.

Becoming aware of other risk factors

Several other factors increase your odds of developing the metabolic syndrome. Some are irreversible, but others are within your control:

- **Postmenopausal status:** The hormones that are secreted while a woman has periods may protect against the development of the metabolic syndrome and explain why cardiovascular disease occurs so much later in females than in males.

- **Tobacco exposure:** Smoking greatly increases the risk for the metabolic syndrome. Unfortunately, exposure to second-hand smoke does as well. In a study published online in the journal *Circulation* in August 2005, the prevalence of the metabolic syndrome was 5.4 percent for adolescents exposed to tobacco and 8.7 percent for adolescents who were active smokers. In overweight adolescents, the risk was 19.6 percent for those exposed to tobacco smoke and 23.6 percent for active smokers.

- **Low socioeconomic status:** Studies of many communities have shown that as socioeconomic status declines, the prevalence of the metabolic syndrome increases. This connection may result from unhealthy food choices and the increased stress associated with low socioeconomic status.

- **High carbohydrate diet:** People who eat lots of carbohydrates, especially *refined* (processed) carbohydrates, tend to have a higher prevalence of the metabolic syndrome. Refined carbohydrates tend to raise your glucose, insulin, and triglyceride levels while lowering your HDL (good) cholesterol. Eating more carbohydrates with low glycemic indexes (which I explain in Chapter 5) can help protect you against the metabolic syndrome.

- **No alcohol consumption:** Surprisingly, people who don't drink any alcohol tend to be more at risk for the metabolic syndrome. Women should drink no more than a glass of wine or its equivalent a night and no more than five glasses a week. Men should drink no more than two glasses of wine a night and no more than ten glasses a week.

- **Mexican-American ethnicity:** The metabolic syndrome is more prevalent in the Mexican-American population. Within that population, it's more prevalent in women than men.

So if you are an overweight Mexican-American female smoker who doesn't drink any alcohol, eats a lot of refined carbohydrates, and is postmenopausal, pick up your telephone now and make an appointment with your doctor!

Recognizing Major Signs and Symptoms

Patients with the metabolic syndrome have a large number of abnormalities, many of which predispose them to heart disease and heart attacks. These abnormalities can be divided into physical signs and symptoms and laboratory abnormalities.

The metabolic syndrome has been defined by several different groups, including the National Cholesterol Education Program and the World Health Organization. To make a diagnosis of the metabolic syndrome, the National Cholesterol Education Program requires the following:

- *Central obesity* (meaning obesity with the fat concentrated around the waist) with a waist circumference of 40 inches in males and 36 inches in females
- Abnormal blood fats, including triglyceride levels greater than 150 mg/dl and HDL cholesterol levels of less than 40 mg/dl in men and less than 50 mg/dl in women
- Blood pressure greater than 130/85
- Fasting blood glucose greater than 110 mg/dl

The requirements of the World Health Organization are slightly different. It identifies insulin resistance (the metabolic syndrome) by one of the following:

- Type 2 diabetes
- Impaired fasting glucose (see Chapter 1)
- Impaired glucose tolerance (see Chapter 1)

plus two of the following:

- Blood pressure greater than or equal to 140/90 (or being on blood pressure medication).
- Triglycerides of 150 mg/dl or greater.
- HDL cholesterol of less than 35 in men or 39 in women.
- BMI greater than 30 kg/m^2 or a ratio of the waist divided by the hip circumference of greater than 0.9 in men and 0.85 in women.
- The excretion of 20 ug/min or more of albumin in the urine. (*Albumin* is a protein found in the blood that normally does not leak into the urine.)

Identifying physical signs and symptoms

The physical signs and symptoms of the metabolic syndrome often overlap with those of prediabetes. They include:

- **High blood pressure:** This symptom may result from the increased levels of insulin in the body, which are necessary to keep the blood glucose normal.

- **Increased abdominal visceral fat:** The waist is greater than 40 inches in men and 35 inches in women.

- **Obesity:** Many, but not all, people with the metabolic syndrome are obese.

- **Sedentary lifestyle:** However, an active lifestyle does not rule out the metabolic syndrome.

- **Polycystic ovarian syndrome:** This group of abnormalities includes menstrual irregularity, infertility, and excess facial and body hair in females that is related to insulin resistance.

- **Thinking disorders and Alzheimer's disease:** Insulin is important in normal brain function, and insulin resistance is associated with thinking disorders like trouble calculating or memory loss as in Alzheimer's disease.

Looking at laboratory abnormalities

People with the metabolic syndrome have a large number of laboratory abnormalities, in addition to those that are part of the definition of the syndrome. These abnormalities contribute to the heart disease that is the outcome of untreated metabolic syndrome. Most of the abnormalities reverse with appropriate treatment.

I realize that this list may make your eyes cross, but please don't get overwhelmed. What follows is pretty technical, but it's crucial information if you get lab work done to test for the metabolic syndrome. Earmark this page so you can return to it after you've had lab work done. That way, you can compare your test results to see whether you have any questions for your doctor or need any clarification of how you've been diagnosed.

The important laboratory abnormalities are

- **Elevated fasting blood glucose and/or impaired glucose tolerance:** Your blood glucose is 100 mg/dl (5.6 mmol/L) or greater after an overnight fast or 140 mg/dl (7.8 mmol/L) or greater after a glucose challenge (see Chapter 10).

- **Elevated blood levels of insulin:** The insulin is produced by your pancreas to overcome the higher levels of blood glucose.

✔ **Blood triglyceride level of 150 mg/dl or greater after you've been fasting:** Your triglyceride levels are usually high after eating (especially after eating carbohydrates), but they should be less than 150 mg/dl after you have fasted overnight.

✔ **Blood HDL-C (good cholesterol) levels of less than or equal to 50 mg/dl in women and less than or equal to 40 mg/dl in men:** Higher levels of HDL-C protect you against heart disease.

✔ **Increased production of small, dense LDL-C particles:** This type of cholesterol particle tends to cause more cardiovascular disease.

✔ **Microalbuminuria:** This term means that lab tests find 20 micrograms/dl or more of albumin in a random urine specimen.

✔ **Reduced levels of testosterone and sex hormone–binding globulin in middle-aged men:** These findings predict the development of the metabolic syndrome. They are early markers for insulin resistance and abnormal glucose metabolism.

✔ **Elevated levels of C-reactive protein (CRP):** This protein in the blood indicates increased inflammation. Exactly how CRP becomes elevated is not clear. Visceral fat tissue may release substances called *cytokines* that cause the release of CRP by the liver, or insulin resistance may be responsible for more cytokines and more CRP.

Inflammation plays an important role in the metabolic syndrome:

- *Ferritin* is another compound associated with inflammation that is found in excess in the metabolic syndrome. When your triglyceride is greater than 149 mg/dl, and when your fasting blood glucose is greater than 100 mg/dl, your ferritin levels are elevated as well.

- Abnormalities in arteries in people with the metabolic syndrome show many inflammatory cells. They may explain the abnormal function of the lining of the arteries that leads to cardiovascular disease.

✔ **Elevated levels of plasminogen activator inhibitor-1 (PAI-1):** PAI-1 blocks the production of plasminogen activator, resulting in decreased plasmin (fibrinolysin). *Plasmin* is the substance that breaks down clots in your blood stream. Having elevated PAI-1 levels tends to increase your chance of getting a blood clot and having a resultant heart attack.

✔ **Elevated levels of uric acid leading to uric acid kidney stones (and gouty arthritis):** The elevation may be related to the increased use of fructose in our diets. Fructose is known to increase uric acid in the blood. People with the metabolic syndrome have very acidic urine, which tends to cause the formation of uric acid stones.

✒ **Elevated blood levels of gamma-glutamyl transpeptidase (GGT):** This enzyme is released from the liver. Its main function is the transfer of amino acids into cells. It has been found to be elevated before the onset of the metabolic syndrome, coronary heart disease, and death. GGT is elevated when your body mass index (BMI), blood pressure, triglycerides, and blood glucose are elevated. This enzyme could be a marker for the future development of the metabolic syndrome.

✒ **Elevated levels of homocysteine:** *Homocysteine* is an amino acid that is made in the body from another amino acid, methionine. Deficiencies of the vitamins folic acid (B9), pyridoxine (B6), and cyanocobalamin (B12) can lead to higher levels of homocysteine. A high level of homocysteine is associated with cardiovascular disease. Homocysteine may do its damage by preventing the formation of the substances that give arteries structure: collagen, elastin, and proteoglycans. So far, attempts to reduce heart disease by lowering homocysteine with vitamins have not been successful.

✒ **Abnormal liver function tests:** This result is probably caused by non-alcoholic fatty liver disease, which is a consequence of the metabolic syndrome. Usually you don't experience signs and symptoms of this disease, but if you do, they include pain in the right side over the liver, an enlarged liver, and increased gallstones. This condition can move on to *cirrhosis,* where the liver is irreversibly damaged.

Could fructose be the culprit?

An important study published in the *American Journal of Physiology-Renal Physiology* in October 2005 suggests that our old friend fructose may be at the heart (pun intended) of the worldwide epidemic of the metabolic syndrome. When fructose was fed to rats, it caused many features of the metabolic syndrome, such as high triglycerides, increased insulin, and high uric acid. Sucrose (table sugar) did not create the same problems. Lowering the uric acid with drugs reversed or prevented the features of the metabolic syndrome. Giving the rats a drug that blocked uric acid production before feeding them fructose prevented elevated insulin levels, elevated blood pressure, elevated triglycerides, and weight gain. Finally, uric acid negatively affected the function of the tissue that lines blood vessels, an effect that would promote cardiovascular disease.

Reversing the Causes of the Metabolic Syndrome

Now that you know how you develop the metabolic syndrome and the major signs and symptoms, you should have a pretty good idea of how to reverse the causes and avoid the consequences (cardiovascular disease). If you take action, not only can you reverse the metabolic syndrome, but you will avoid or reverse prediabetes at the same time. You can kill two birds with one stone (while ensuring that you will be around to throw many more stones in the future).

The harder you work, the less likely you will suffer from the consequences of cardiovascular disease and heart attacks. For details about how to make these changes, be sure to read Part V of this book:

✔ **Lose weight:** If one or both of your parents have the metabolic syndrome, do whatever you can to avoid having a body mass index of 25 or greater. In fact, try to have a BMI on the low side of normal, around 20. As I point out earlier in the chapter, even high normal BMIs are associated with features of the metabolic syndrome. Losing weight will reduce your blood glucose, your blood pressure, your total and bad cholesterol, and your triglycerides.

If you are at risk for the metabolic syndrome and you have children, take action now to make sure they are never overweight!

✔ **Get active:** Start walking for at least 30 minutes daily, and preferably for an hour. Make the time (see Chapter 7 for pointers). And do little things throughout your day to increase your activity level:

   • Leave your car at home whenever possible.

   • Park your car blocks from your destination so you're forced to walk the remaining distance. (You may find it easier to locate a parking space this way, which will also lower your stress level!)

   • Walk up stairs instead of taking the elevator.

   • Wear a pedometer and keep a record of the number of steps you walk each day. Try to add a few hundred steps whenever possible.

   • Take a walk during your lunch break.

✔ **Stop smoking:** I know it's easy to say and hard to do, but you simply must do it. And you also must demand that nobody smoke in your environment. Second-hand smoke greatly increases the risk for the metabolic syndrome.

✔ **Eat fewer refined carbohydrates:** Eat fewer carbohydrates period, and when you do eat them, focus on unrefined, low glycemic carbs (see Chapter 5).

✔ **Skip the diet soda:** An April 2009 article in *Diabetes Care* showed that people who drank diet soda at least daily had a significantly greater risk of developing the metabolic syndrome and type 2 diabetes. The exact connection is unclear.

✔ **Drink a bit of alcohol:** If you're a recovered alcoholic, obviously you need to skip this advice. For everyone else, research shows that a glass of wine each night may do you some good. But don't overdo it! Too much alcohol ruins your liver and does a lot of other damage. A November 2008 article in the *Journal of Clinical Endocrinology & Metabolism* showed that excess drinking also increases your risk for developing the features of the metabolic syndrome — exactly what you don't want!

✔ **Follow the Dietary Approaches to Stop Hypertension (DASH) diet:** The DASH diet, which was developed to treat high blood pressure, has also been shown to be valuable in the metabolic syndrome. Following the DASH diet, which involves increasing your intake of fruits and vegetables, results in higher HDL cholesterol, lower triglycerides, lower blood pressure, reduced weight, and lower blood glucose.

Dealing with Uncontrolled Metabolic Syndrome

If you haven't been able to prevent the metabolic syndrome, you can at least minimize the damage by treating some of the consequences. Each of the topics I introduce here gets more attention in Part V.

Reversing high blood glucose

As I explain in Chapter 18, numerous drugs are available to lower high blood glucose levels (*hyperglycemia*). Their use depends on the severity of your situation. Some of the drugs that can be used include the following:

✔ **Metformin:** This drug affects the liver in order to reduce the release of glucose, thus lowering your blood glucose. It can reverse some of the features of the metabolic syndrome.

✔ **Actos:** This drug actually increases insulin sensitivity. However, it has other side effects like water retention that make its use problematic.

✔ **Acarbose:** This drug slows the breakdown of complex carbohydrates in your intestine so the uptake of glucose is reduced. However, patients complain of abdominal discomfort due to gas when the bacteria in the lower intestine ingest the carbohydrate.

If drugs aren't effective, you may want to consider bariatric surgery to achieve significant weight loss (see Chapter 19). Bariatric surgery can reverse all the features of the metabolic syndrome and maintain the reversal for more than ten years.

Lowering your blood pressure

Numerous medications are available that can lower your blood pressure, but experts recommend a drug from the class called *Angiotensin-Converting Enzyme (ACE) inhibitors* that have been shown to be especially protective of the kidneys while they lower the blood pressure. If this medication is not effective alone, your doctor may recommend adding a diuretic, which causes water loss.

Improving your blood fats

Many drugs may be helpful here as well. Among them are

- ✔ **Statin drugs:** They lower your total and bad cholesterol and may raise your good cholesterol.
- ✔ **Niacin:** It can raise your HDL-C (good cholesterol), but it also raises blood glucose.
- ✔ **Fibrates:** These are very helpful in the treatment of elevated triglycerides.

After you have the metabolic syndrome, you can take many steps to combat it. But as with every other disease, an ounce of prevention is worth a pound of cure. Don't let yourself get to the stage where you need these medications or even surgery.

As I note earlier in the chapter, growing evidence indicates that insulin resistance, the basis for the metabolic syndrome, may play a major role in Alzheimer's disease. Making lifestyle changes now, which will slow down or reverse the metabolic syndrome and prediabetes, may do the same for Alzheimer's disease. What are you waiting for?

Chapter 10

The Testing Spectrum: Having Essential Tests and Interpreting Results

*T*o figure out if you have prediabetes, or to figure out whether you're getting it under control after you've been diagnosed, you need to be prepared to have a few essential lab tests, all of which I cover in this chapter.

If you truly despise making the trip to the lab, scientists have devised highly accurate home test kits that save you the trouble. With just a drop or two of your blood, you can get test results from a mail-in lab service.

And honestly, some of the most important numbers you need to know don't require any blood work at all. Instead, they're basic measurements like height, weight, waist circumference, and blood pressure. With the exception of blood pressure, I don't discuss these measurements in this chapter. But that's not a commentary on their importance — just a vote of confidence in your ability to wield a tape measure and a bathroom scale.

Checking Your Blood Glucose Level

The foundation of a diagnosis of prediabetes is your blood glucose level. This first and most essential test must be done correctly.

Going to a lab: Fasting glucose or glucose challenge

As I explain way back in Chapter 1, prediabetes is defined by the level of glucose in your blood, either after you've fasted overnight or two hours after you've eaten 75 grams of glucose. Because this test result has such important consequences for your health, it must be highly accurate. At the moment, that level of accuracy is achievable only in a clinical laboratory.

If you and your doctor suspect that you have prediabetes, your doctor will give you a laboratory slip and ask you to go to the lab after an overnight fast (because this is the simplest way to perform the test). The lab tech will put a needle into your vein and withdraw a blood specimen. Here are some key results:

✔ If your blood glucose is between 100 and 125 mg/dl (5.6–6.9 mmol/L) on more than one occasion, you have prediabetes.

✔ If your blood glucose is at or above 126 mg/dl (7 mmol/L) on more than one occasion, you have diabetes.

Some doctors believe that your response to a *glucose challenge* is a more accurate measure of abnormal metabolism than a fasting test. For a glucose challenge, your doctor gives you 75 grams of glucose to drink and sends you to the laboratory two hours after you've consumed the drink. The crucial results of this test are as follows:

✔ If, on more than one occasion, your blood glucose is 140–199 mg/dl (7.8–11.0 mmol/L) two hours after consuming 75 grams of glucose, you have prediabetes.

✔ If, on more than one occasion, your blood glucose is at or above 200 mg/dl (11.1 mmol/L) two hours after consuming 75 grams of glucose, you have diabetes.

Don't do a lot of exercise before the fasting test, and don't fast or change your diet before the glucose challenge. Any of these changes to your routine will make the test results inaccurate.

Using your own meter at home

Let's say you do have prediabetes. What then? Your next step is to get your own glucose meter and do a little glucose testing at home. You don't have to test as regularly as you would with diabetes, but knowing your blood glucose can be very valuable.

In the next section, I offer some advice to help you choose among the many home meters available. First, I want to make sure that you do the test properly no matter which meter you use.

How does the meter work?

Two kinds of meters are on the market today. Both use a test strip that has an enzyme in it that reacts with the glucose in your blood. One type of strip becomes colored by the reaction, and the meter reads the color. The other type of strip produces electrons, and the meter converts the amount of electrons into a glucose reading.

How frequently should you test?

With prediabetes, how often you test is pretty much up to you, but here are two suggestions:

✔ Once a week, take a fasting blood glucose reading after an overnight fast. See if your treatment program has helped you get below the magic number of 100 mg/dl.

✔ Also use the meter to find out what different kinds of foods do to your blood glucose. If a given food raises your blood glucose to more than 140 mg/dl one hour after eating it, consider reducing your consumption of that food in the future. You may be able to keep enjoying that food, but you at least need to reduce the portion.

How do you do the test?

The specific answer depends on the meter you're using. However, the test is basically done in the following way:

1. **Put a *lancet* (a sharp needle) in its device and cock the device.**

2. **Turn on your meter.** If you are using a meter with a drum, a test strip will drop down from inside the meter. If you have to insert the test strip, doing so will usually turn on the meter.

3. **Wait for the beep that tells you the strip is ready for testing.**

4. **Test on a clean finger.** (You don't have to wipe the finger with alcohol.) Put the side of your finger against the opening in the lancet device.

5. **Press the button that releases the lancet against the side of your finger.**

6. **As a drop of blood forms, hold it against the end of the test strip.**

7. **Wait for the beep that tells you there is enough blood on the strip.**

8. **If the test strip doesn't have enough blood, squeeze your finger a little more and add blood.**

9. **Within a few seconds, you should have a result.**

Here are a few tips to make testing more accurate and safe:

- You should never use your lancets on anyone else.

- You also shouldn't use your meter for anyone else. The reason for this is that you may want to show your doctor your test results, and you don't want to confuse them with someone else's.

- You don't have to get the blood from your finger. If you get blood from another part of your body, the result should still be accurate *except* within a half hour after exercise and within an hour after eating.

- You need to always keep your vial of test strips closed. Loose test strips in a vial deteriorate rapidly if the vial is open.

- To increase the flow of blood, you can put a tight rubber band around your finger where it meets your hand.

- You want to check whether your meter reports test results in *whole blood* or in *plasma.* Clinical labs always report plasma levels, and all doctors' recommendations are in plasma levels. (The blood glucose level of whole blood is 12 percent lower than a plasma blood glucose.)

Choosing a blood glucose meter

Meters are relatively inexpensive, and many manufacturers give them away so you have to buy their strips. Strips are not interchangeable between meters, so you have to buy the strips made for your specific machine.

Try to get a new meter every year or two because they change so rapidly and they are so inexpensive. Test strips usually cost about $1 per test, regardless of the meter you use.

Your meter needs to have a memory that records the time and date that you take the test, as well as a way of downloading the test results to a computer for evaluation and storage.

You can choose among four major manufacturers of glucose meters for home testing: Abbott Diabetes Care, Bayer Diagnostics, LifeScan, and Roche Diagnostics. Each company offers numerous glucose meters. Table 10-1 shows the features of one meter from each company. If you need a special feature, such as a verbal announcement of the glucose reading, you can shop according to that special need.

Table 10-1		Comparing Glucose Meters			
Manufacturer	*Meter Name*	*Sample Size (Micro-liters)*	*Time of Test (Seconds)*	*Name of Strips*	*Multi-site Testing?*
Abbott	Free-Style Lite	0.3	5	Free-Style Lite	Yes
Bayer	Breeze2	1.0	5	Breeze2	Yes
LifeScan	One-Touch Ultra	1.0	5	One-Touch Ultra	Yes
Roche	Accu-Chek Compact Plus	1.5	5	Compact Plus	Yes

As you can see, the differences among the various meters are slight. The Abbott meter uses the least blood, so if you have trouble getting a sample, that meter may be best for you. All these meters can remember hundreds of tests and download them to a computer. The Bayer meter uses a 10-test disc, and the Roche meter uses a 17-test drum, so using them is a little more convenient. The Abbott and LifeScan meters are smaller than the other two, which may be a reason to buy one of them.

Your doctor and/or insurance company may prefer a particular meter, so consider those possibilities before you buy.

Tracking Your Glucose for the Last 90 Days

Single tests of your blood glucose are very useful to know what's happening at any given second. But what about the other 86,399 seconds in a day? Your blood glucose can vary greatly in a few minutes, especially after you've eaten or exercised. What you need is a test that can tell you how your blood glucose has been doing for a significant length of time. The *hemoglobin A1c* is that test.

The basis of the test is that *hemoglobin,* a substance found in red blood cells that carries oxygen from the lungs to all cells in the body, forms an irreversible compound called *glycated hemoglobin* or *glycohemoglobin* when in the presence of glucose. The more glucose you have in your blood, the more glycated hemoglobin will be formed. The attachment occurs in different ways called *A1a, A1b,* and *A1c.* The A1c makes up two-thirds of the glycated hemoglobin and is easiest to measure.

Your hemoglobin is packed into your red blood cells, which last for 60 to 90 days. As a result, when you have a blood sample taken and your red blood cells are broken open, the hemoglobin A1c reflects your level of blood glucose for the last 60 to 90 days — instead of the last second, minute, or hour.

In people with normal blood glucose levels, the hemoglobin A1c is between 4 to 6 percent of their total hemoglobin. As your blood glucose levels rise, so does your hemoglobin A1c. In general, if your hemoglobin A1c is kept below 7 percent, you don't develop the complications of diabetes that I discuss in Chapter 13. (The 7 percent marker is the standard of the American Diabetes Association. Other organizations prefer a hemoglobin A1c of less than 6.5 percent.)

Because hemoglobin A1c reflects your average blood glucose for the last 60 to 90 days, scientists can create a chart that tells you what the average blood glucose level is for any level of hemoglobin A1c. For example, a normal hemoglobin A1c of 6 percent corresponds to an average plasma glucose of 140 mg/dl. A hemoglobin A1c of 7 percent corresponds to an average plasma glucose of 170 mg/dl, and a hemoglobin A1c of 8 percent corresponds to an average plasma glucose of 210 mg/dl.

In the future, hemoglobin A1c test results will be provided along with their corresponding plasma glucose numbers and referred to as someone's *average blood glucose.* That's because doctors and patients are used to thinking in terms of blood glucose levels.

A hemoglobin A1c between 6 and 7 percent corresponds with the blood glucose levels found in prediabetes. You want to get yours below 6 percent by making lifestyle changes.

The hemoglobin A1c test is not used to diagnose diabetes at this time because there is too much variation among laboratories; labs use different test methods, and opinions differ as to what is normal and what is not. When the test becomes more standardized, it will undoubtedly be used to make the diagnosis.

However, in a few situations the hemoglobin A1c test is not accurate:

- When a patient has anemia, the decrease in red blood cells results in a falsely low hemoglobin A1c.

- Patients with a hereditary disease of the red blood cells called a *hemoglobinopathy* also give a falsely low result.

- Using supplements like vitamins C and E alter the result in a downward direction.

- Liver disease and kidney disease inaccurately lower the hemoglobin A1c.

- The use of salicylates like aspirin can lower your hemoglobin A1c (but not the small dose recommended by doctors to prevent heart attacks).

Knowing Your Cholesterol Levels

Abnormal levels of cholesterol contribute to heart disease in prediabetes and diabetes, as well as to the metabolic syndrome (which I discuss in Chapter 9). Just knowing your total cholesterol is not enough. The significance of the cholesterol depends upon how much of it is *good* cholesterol (HDL-C) and *bad* cholesterol (LDL-C). You also need to know your level of *triglycerides:* another type of fat that may do damage to your heart if the levels are too high.

Recognizing four kinds of lipoproteins

Because cholesterol is not soluble in water, it has to be packaged into fat particles called *lipoproteins*. These particles have protein on the outside and fat on the inside. In this way, they can be transported throughout the body. Your body has four different types of lipoproteins:

- ✔ *Chylomicrons* are the largest of the fat particles. When fat is absorbed from the intestine, it is packed into chylomicrons that are rapidly cleared from the blood. Chylomicrons do not cause cardiovascular disease.

- ✔ *Very low-density lipoprotein (VLDL)* particles are smaller than chylomicrons and contain mostly triglycerides. Triglyceride is the main fat that makes up vegetable oil and animal fats. (The other fat in these products is cholesterol.) VLDL particles also don't contribute to cardiovascular disease but just act as carriers.

- ✔ *High-density lipoprotein (HDL)* particles are smaller than VLDL particles. HDL is called "good cholesterol" because these particles help to clear the arteries of cholesterol and prevent cardiovascular disease.

- ✔ *Low-density lipoprotein (LDL)* is the smallest particle. Dubbed "bad cholesterol," LDL carries cholesterol to the arteries and deposits it there, causing increased cardiovascular disease.

If you are being treated for having abnormal blood fats, your doctor should run a *fasting lipid panel* (which tests for HDL, LDL, total cholesterol, and triglycerides) once a year or more often.

Table 10-2 shows the recommended levels for these various fat particles.

Table 10-2 Levels of Fat and the Risk for Coronary Artery Disease

Risk	LDL Cholesterol (mg/dl)	HDL Cholesterol (mg/dl)	Triglycerides (mg/dl)
Higher	Greater than 130	Less than 35	Greater than 400
Borderline	100 to 129	35 to 45	150 to 399
Lower	Less than 100	Greater than 45	Less than 150

The risk of heart disease increases as your HDL cholesterol decreases. Observation of the citizens of Framingham, Massachusetts over many decades showed that when the total cholesterol is divided by the good cholesterol, if the result is less than 4.5, the risk of a heart attack is reduced.

LDL cholesterol is also very important. A study in *The New England Journal of Medicine* in March 2004 using a drug to lower LDL cholesterol (atorvastatin) showed that participants experienced a significant reduction in heart attacks when their LDL cholesterol was reduced to 62 mg/dl compared to reducing it to 95 mg/dl. (Before this study, just getting a patient's LDL under 100 mg/dl was considered excellent treatment.)

If you have the metabolic syndrome (see Chapter 9), having low HDL and high triglycerides is associated with increased heart disease. Treating this syndrome requires raising your HDL and lowering your triglycerides with appropriate drugs.

Deciding whether treatment is necessary

The decision to treat your blood fats is based not only on your levels of the various fats but on the level of your risk to have a heart attack. Here are the three levels of risk:

✔ **Highest:** You have already had vascular disease, such as a stroke, a heart attack, or arterial disease of the legs.

✔ **High:** You fit in this category if you

- Are a male over 45
- Are a female over 55
- Smoke cigarettes
- Have high blood pressure
- Have HDL-C below 35
- Have a father or brother who had a heart attack before age 55
- Have a mother or sister who had a heart attack before age 65
- Have a body mass index over 30

✔ **Low:** You have none of the preceding risk factors.

After you figure out whether your risk is high or low, you and your doctor can decide whether to treat your blood fats and how to treat them based on the recommendations shown in Table 10-3.

Table 10-3   Blood Fats Treatment Based on Your Risk Category

Risk	*Dietary Treatment Alone If Your LDL Is Between*	*Dietary and Drug Treatment If Your LDL Is Greater Than*
Low	160–189	190
High	130–159	160
Very high		100

Treating elevated fat levels with medication

If you and your doctor decide to treat your blood fat levels with medications (as well as with lifestyle changes, such as weight loss), many types of drugs are available. For example,

- *Statin drugs* lower your LDL cholesterol and triglycerides and raise your HDL cholesterol.

- *Nicotinic acid* lowers your LDL-C and triglycerides and raises your HDL-C.

- *Fibric acids* lower your LDL-C and triglycerides while raising your HDL-C.

- *Bile acid sequestrants* lower your LDL-C and raise your HDL-C but don't change the triglycerides.

Keeping Your Blood Pressure in Check

The prevalence of high blood pressure is rising in step with prediabetes and diabetes, and for the same reasons: increased weight and our sedentary lifestyle. This fact is true for every age group.

But even if you've had your blood pressure taken hundreds of times before, do you actually know what the numbers mean? If you're concerned about high blood pressure but don't know what "high" actually means (or what numbers you should be aiming for), keep reading.

Clarifying the numbers

When someone checks your blood pressure, the result looks like this: 120/70. What do the two numbers mean?

- The upper (higher) number is called the *systolic blood pressure* and represents the force with which your heart expels blood into your arteries.

- The lower (smaller) number is the *diastolic blood pressure* and represents the pressure in your arteries when your heart rests for a moment. Before that number can go lower, your heart begins to pump forcefully again.

A blood pressure below 140/90 is considered normal, even for a person with prediabetes. However, if you have diabetes, your goal should be a blood pressure under 130/80. That's because if your heart pumps at a continuously high pressure, it does damage to your arteries (as well as to the heart itself).

Dealing with high blood pressure

As with prediabetes, lifestyle change focused on weight loss and exercise is the cornerstone of treating high blood pressure. You can take a number of steps before resorting to medications. Techniques like meditation and yoga have proved very helpful in lowering blood pressure.

If these measures fail, drug treatment can usually control your blood pressure. The numerous drugs available for treating high blood pressure fall into a few classes:

- ✔ *Diuretics* lower blood pressure by reducing the salt and water in your body. After a while, however, this effect declines, and diuretics then work by reducing the resistance to blood flow in your arteries. Diuretics should be your drug of first choice unless your situation specifically calls for another treatment. These drugs have clearly been shown to reduce illness and death associated with high blood pressure. Examples of diuretics in common use are hydrochlorothiazide and furosemide.

- ✔ Beta-adrenergic receptor blockers, known as *beta blockers,* come next in effectiveness. They act on your blood pressure by reducing the forcefulness of your heart while reducing the release of renin and angiotensin, hormones that tend to raise your blood pressure. They slow your heart, so if you need to have your heart speed up (for example during exercise), you may not do well with these drugs. Examples are propranolol and metoprolol.

- ✔ *Calcium channel blocking agents* relax the muscles that contract to make your arteries smaller. This action lowers your blood pressure. These agents are added on when the two previous classes of drugs don't work. Commonly used varieties are verapamil and nifedipine.

- ✔ *Angiotensin-converting enzyme (ACE) inhibitors* block the activity of an enzyme that produces a very powerful blood pressure–raising chemical called *angiotensin II.* These drugs slow the progression of heart failure, kidney disease, and diabetes. They are often used as the drug of first choice when a patient has diabetes and high blood pressure because ACE inhibitors protect the kidneys. Examples are Enalapril and lisinopril.

- ✔ *Angiotensin II receptor blockers* work to lower blood pressure by not allowing the attachment of angiotensin II where it does its work of contracting your arteries. These drugs are similar in action to the ACE inhibitors and, like the ACE inhibitors, protect your kidneys from diabetes. Examples are candesartan and irbesartan.

For a much more extensive discussion of these drugs, see my book *High Blood Pressure For Dummies,* 2nd Edition (Wiley).

Most high blood pressure should be treated first with a diuretic. If the diuretic doesn't control your blood pressure, a beta blocker is added. Next would be a calcium channel blocker or an ACE inhibitor.

Looking for Evidence of Inflammation

Inflammation plays a large role in prediabetes and diabetes, so looking for the presence of inflammation may help evaluate the severity of your condition. The Cardiovascular Health Study (an ongoing study of people over age 65) has found that people with high levels of C-reactive protein are twice as likely to develop diabetes as those with normal levels. C-reactive protein (CRP) reflects the amount of inflammation in your body. As I note in Chapter 9, your CRP level is elevated if you have the metabolic syndrome, which is a precursor for cardiovascular disease.

The question is whether CRP is just a marker for heart disease or whether it actually plays a role in the development of heart disease. Two studies in *The New England Journal of Medicine* in January 2005 suggest that CRP may actually cause heart disease:

- ✔ In the first study, patients took high doses of the statin drugs, which lower both cholesterol and CRP. Participants were then followed for the development of heart attacks and death. Patients whose CRP was lowered, regardless of whether their LDL (bad) cholesterol went down, experienced a significant reduction in heart attacks and death.

- ✔ In the other study, patients were treated with moderate and intensive statin therapy. Intensive therapy slowed the development of cardiovascular disease. Patients with lower CRP levels had slower progression even when their cholesterol was the same as patients with higher CRP levels.

Testing CRP levels is especially helpful for people at high risk for a heart attack. (You can determine your level of risk by looking at the section "Deciding if treatment is necessary" earlier in this chapter.)

CRP is a blood test, and a highly sensitive version of the test is now available. Here's how the test results indicate your risk for developing cardiovascular disease, according to the American Heart Association:

- ✔ Your risk is low if your CRP is lower than 1.0 mg/L.

- ✔ Your risk is average if your CRP is between 1.0 and 3.0 mg/L.

- ✔ Your risk is high if your CRP is higher than 3.0 mg/L.

People who are at high risk for cardiovascular disease should be treated intensively to lower their blood pressure, cholesterol, weight, and so forth. They must also be encouraged to quit smoking. All these changes can lower your CRP levels.

Other tests for inflammation exist (such as the *erythrocyte sedimentation rate,* a measure of how fast your blood settles in a tube) but have not been proven very helpful.

Hunting for Nutrient Deficiencies

In addition to water and sources of energy like carbohydrate, fat, and protein, your body needs a variety of vitamins and minerals for good health. Fortunately, in the United States, most people get sufficient quantities of these substances in the food they eat. But there are exceptions, which I point out below.

Keeping your vitamin levels on target

You need a large number of vitamins in tiny quantities for good health. Table 10-4 lists the vitamins, their function, and the food sources that provide the largest amounts of them.

You can get most of these vitamins in the foods you eat, but specific diseases may correspond to a deficiency of each of the vitamins. See the book *Vitamins For Dummies* by Christopher Hobbs and Elson Haas (Wiley) for more information. If you and your doctor suspect that you may have a specific vitamin deficiency, you can have lab work done to check your blood levels of all these vitamins.

The one vitamin that should probably be measured much more frequently than all others is vitamin D. Scientists have found that vitamin D does a lot more than just help with absorption of calcium. Vitamin D is now considered similar to a hormone because it has effects all over the body. For example, vitamin D may protect against the following conditions:

- Alzheimer's disease
- Autoimmune arthritis
- Cancer of the large intestine and breast
- Cardiovascular disease
- Diabetes
- Multiple sclerosis
- Stroke

Table 10-4	Vitamins You Need	
Vitamin	*Function*	*Food Source*
Vitamin A	Needed for healthy skin and bones	Milk and green vegetables
Vitamin B₁ (thiamin)	Converts carbohydrates into energy	Meat and whole grain cereals
Vitamin B₂ (riboflavin)	Needed to use food properly	Milk, cheese, fish, and green vegetables
Vitamin B₆ (pyridox-ine), pantothenic acid, and biotin	All needed for growth	Liver, yeast, and many other foods
Vitamin B₁₂	Keeps the red blood cells and the nervous system healthy	Animal foods (for example, meat)
Folic acid	Keeps the red blood cells and the nervous system healthy	Green vegetables
Niacin	Helps release energy	Lean meat, fish, nuts, and legumes
Vitamin C	Helps maintain supportive tissues	Fruit and potatoes
Vitamin D	Helps with absorption of calcium, plus many other functions.	Dairy products, and it is made in the skin when exposed to sunlight
Vitamin E	Helps maintain cells	Vegetable oils and whole grain cereals
Vitamin K	Needed for proper clotting of the blood	Leafy vegetables, and it is made by bacteria in your intestine

Make sure you are getting enough vitamin D by having your doctor measure *25 hydroxy vitamin D.* Your level should be greater than 30 ng/ml. If not, you can take supplemental vitamin D by mouth.

Stocking up on minerals

Many minerals are also essential for good health. Table 10-5 lists the minerals, what they do, and how to obtain adequate amounts.

Table 10-5	Minerals You Need	
Mineral	*Function*	*Food Source*
Calcium	For bones and teeth	Dairy
Phosphorus	For bones and teeth	Dairy
Magnesium	For bones and teeth	Dairy
Iron	Hemoglobin in red blood cells	Meat
Sodium	Regulates body water	Salt
Chromium	Stimulates fatty acids and cholesterol for brain function	Beef, liver, eggs
Iodine	For thyroid hormone	Salt, bread
Chlorine, cobalt, tin, zinc	Various functions	Lean meat, fish, nuts, and legumes

Your levels of these minerals can be measured, and you can take mineral supplements if necessary.

Getting a TSH test

The thyroid-stimulating hormone (TSH) test is a screening test for thyroid disease. Because thyroid disease often accompanies diabetes and thyroid disease tends to be asymptomatic, a TSH test is a good idea beginning at age 35. The test is also done on newborns to screen for low thyroid function. Prompt treatment with thyroid hormone can prevent loss of brain function. The test is done by measuring the TSH in a blood sample.

Chapter 11

Children and the Elderly: Special Considerations

*M*uch of what I write in the rest of this book applies to all people, young and old alike. So why do I devote a special chapter to children and the elderly? The reasons are different for each:

✔ Children are growing and in a constant state of change. If that change involves putting on too much weight, the potential for future harm is great. Kids have a long time to develop complications if they progress to diabetes.

✔ The elderly have various medical conditions that complicate their health. Plus, they may have memory and learning problems that make caring for them more difficult.

If your child is putting on excess weight, take some of the steps I suggest in this chapter to reverse the situation as early as you can. Dealing with a few extra pounds early on is much easier than reversing a large weight gain that has been present for several years.

If you are elderly (over 70 years of age) or have an elderly parent, keep in mind that just growing older makes you more insulin resistant and more subject to prediabetes and diabetes. The suggestions in this chapter can help you delay or prevent the transition from prediabetes to diabetes and perhaps even return to the state of normal blood glucose metabolism.

Diagnosing and Managing Prediabetes in Children

Childhood obesity experts are discovering signs of diabetes, high blood pressure, high cholesterol, and liver disease in many children under the age of 12. The result may be a whole generation of kids who will have a lower life expectancy than earlier generations.

More than 15 percent of children and adolescents (from age 6 to 19) are overweight in the United States. This percentage has doubled since the 1970s. The body mass index, which I explain in Chapter 6, is a reasonable measure to identify children who are overweight. Children who are overweight at age 8 are at risk of becoming overweight adults.

Before you concern yourself with reversing prediabetes or preventing type 2 diabetes in your child, you need to know if she is overweight or obese. If you determine that she is, you want to know what to do. I cover these subjects in this section.

Checking if your child is overweight

In Chapter 6, I show you how to calculate your body mass index (BMI). For children, determining whether the BMI is a problem is more complex than for adults. That's because children are growing and may possibly grow out of the problem.

Children with a BMI from the 5th to the 84th percentile are considered normal in weight. Children are considered at risk for being overweight if their BMI is between the 85th and 94th percentile for height and weight. Obesity is defined as a BMI at or above the 95th percentile for height and weight.

The easiest way to determine whether your child's BMI is a cause of concern is to use the calculator at http://kidshealth.org/parent/food/weight/bmi_charts.html. You plug in your child's gender, date of birth, height, and weight. The calculator works for children age 2 to 20. It calculates the BMI and then tells you how that BMI compares to healthy children of the same age, sex, and height. Don't think in terms of normal BMIs for adults. BMIs that may appear to be normal in adults may be in the overweight category for a child who is shorter than an adult.

If your child is in the overweight category, she may grow out of it as she gets older and taller. But she may not, which means that some change in her lifestyle is necessary. Your job is to check her BMI regularly over time to see if it gets better or worse. That information can help you determine what action to take.

If your child is obese, you don't have the luxury of taking a wait-and-see approach. You must encourage lifestyle changes immediately.

Securing a diagnosis and taking action

For a child who is obese or who remains overweight, you need to find out whether prediabetes is present. When you get a diagnosis, the next step is to create an action plan. I cover both topics here.

Making the diagnosis in children

You must find out if your overweight or obese child has prediabetes already. The diagnosis is made the same way as it is for adults: by doing a *fasting blood glucose* test or a *glucose challenge*:

- ✔ **Fasting blood glucose:** The lab checks your child's blood glucose levels after an overnight fast. A healthy child's test results will be less than 100 mg/dl.

- ✔ **Glucose challenge:** The lab checks your child's blood glucose two hours after he or she consumes a calculated amount of glucose. The test results should be less than 140 mg/dl.

  How much glucose does your child consume for this test? For each kilogram of body weight, he drinks 1.75 grams of glucose. Let's say your child weighs 60 pounds. Your pediatrician divides that number by 2.2 to get the number of kilograms, which in this case is 27.3. Then he multiplies that number by 1.75. He knows to give your child 47.8 (or approximately 48) grams of glucose.

Many experts believe that the fasting blood glucose test misses too many children with prediabetes, and they prefer using the glucose challenge.

Some doctors also suggest that the hemoglobin A1c test, which I describe in Chapter 10, should be used to diagnose prediabetes in children. A hemoglobin A1c of 6 to 6.5 percent would be considered diagnostic of prediabetes. (A result of 6 percent corresponds to an average blood glucose level of 140 mg/dl.)

Planning a lifestyle program

If your child has been diagnosed with prediabetes, what do you do next? I make several recommendations in Chapters 6 and 9, which I discuss at greater length in Part V. But this list will get you started:

- ✔ **Get your child's buy-in.** Sit down and discuss with your child why it's necessary to make some changes in his exercise and eating habits in order to prevent future illness. This step is crucial because if your child is not on the same page as you, you will meet with all kinds of resistance.

✔ **Begin a daily exercise program with your child.** Don't just direct your child to run and stand there with a stopwatch. What's good for him will be good for you and good for your relationship. The eventual goal should be at least 30 minutes of fairly vigorous exercise every day, as I describe in Chapter 17. Even better would be a daily regimen of one hour. Include some resistance exercise (as shown in Chapter 17) three days a week.

✔ **Keep screen time under control.** Limit your child to two hours of looking at screens daily, which includes TV, computers, cell phones, video games, and so on. I'm not talking about time spent on the computer doing homework; that time can be excluded from the two-hour limit. I'm talking about nonessential screen time (although what you define as nonessential and what your child defines as nonessential may differ considerably).

✔ **Stop going to fast food restaurants and to restaurants that offer buffets.** You may be able to return to those places after the problem is brought under control, but stay away for now.

✔ **Reduce the amount of animal protein in your child's diet.** Limit it to 3 ounces a day, and substitute vegetable protein like soy and beans when possible. All animal protein, especially meat, carries saturated fats that promote obesity.

✔ **Eliminate processed meats completely.** This includes salami and other luncheon meats, which are filled with chemicals that make people sick over time.

✔ **Try to introduce a variety of vegetables and fruits as early as possible.** The earlier you do so, the more likely your child will eat and enjoy fruits and vegetables. Here are some specific ideas:

  • Get fruits and vegetables into foods your child already likes, like shakes, muffins, lasagna, soup, and omelets.

  • Switch from soda to 100 percent fruit drinks.

  • Mix fruit with yogurt or your child's cereal.

  • Make a snack of raisins, other pieces of dried fruit, and nuts.

  • Serve vegetables as a stir-fry, made with minimal oil.

  • Start a vegetable garden with your child to enjoy the freshest possible produce.

  • Go to a local farmers' market and let your child pick out the vegetables he wants to eat.

  • Start thinking of corn, potatoes, and rice as starches rather than vegetables. Your child should eat less of them.

  • Eat plenty of vegetables yourself. Your child will want to imitate you.

For a toddler, a serving of vegetables is much smaller than for an adult. The serving size is a tablespoon per year of age, so a 5 year old needs just 5 tablespoons per day (not five zucchinis). Past the age of 8, a serving size is a cup of raw vegetables, a half cup of cooked vegetables, or a whole fruit.

Treating your child if lifestyle change fails

If helping your child change her eating and exercise habits does not halt or reverse her prediabetes, you have other options:

✔ **Medications:** I discuss medications for prediabetes in Chapter 4. As yet, the FDA has not approved any medications specifically for prediabetes, but some medications can prevent prediabetes from becoming diabetes. Among the best are metformin, Acarbose, and pioglitazone.

✔ **Bariatric surgery:** Surgery for obesity and to prevent diabetes in children may seem like an extreme solution, but if your child doesn't respond to lifestyle changes or medication, surgery is a good alternative. The surgery is usually done when the child is an adolescent.

The current recommendation is that any adolescent who has a BMI of 35 or higher *plus* any disease risks associated with obesity should be considered for surgery. Also, any adolescent with a BMI of 40 or above, regardless of the presence of other disease risks, should be considered for surgery. The disease risks include:

- Prediabetes or diabetes
- High blood pressure
- Liver abnormalities
- Sleep apnea
- Joint disease

Studies of many adolescents who have undergone bariatric surgery (which I describe in detail in Chapter 19) have determined that the surgery does carry a certain risk. Some children who undergo the less traumatic gastric banding operation experience slipping of the gastric band and some nutrient deficiencies. The more invasive gastric bypass has been associated with pulmonary embolus, shock, intestinal obstruction, postoperative bleeding, and severe malnutrition. You have to weigh the benefits against the risks, but for many children, the benefits far outweigh the risks.

Bariatric surgery does reverse prediabetes, diabetes, high blood pressure, and abnormal cholesterol levels in children. I believe that the gastric bypass operation is superior to the gastric band for control of obesity in adolescents.

Community-wide "thin living"

In 2004, communities throughout France launched an initiative called "Together, Let's Prevent Obesity in Children." (The program acronym is EPODE, which represents the French words for this title.) The initiative was based on a successful program begun in two French towns between 1992 and 1997. The towns followed a healthy nutritional program to change children's eating habits. The initiative included special lessons in schools and colleges, the distribution of breakfasts, physician support, teacher instruction on how to add healthy eating to the curriculum, and school visits by dietitians. Children in these two towns did not gain abnormal amounts of weight compared to other nearby towns, where they did. Families improved their eating habits.

The much larger program begun in 2004 initially included ten towns. Later, that number grew to 113 towns. The towns received suggestions for activities, diets, and community initiatives. Handouts were provided in shops and supermarkets. The towns created safe routes to walk to school, food professionals talked in the schools, and schools encouraged their students to exercise.

The results of the larger program have been encouraging. Obesity levels have fallen. Children are eating more nutritious food, and they are doing more exercise. The program is spreading to communities in Spain, Belgium, and other countries through the European Public Health Alliance.

This kind of community-wide program may be more successful in the long run than individual attempts to reduce obesity and improve food and exercise habits.

Paying Close Attention to the Elderly

George Bernard Shaw was once showing a friend a bust of himself that had been sculpted by the great painter Renoir. Shaw remarked, "It's a funny thing about that bust. As time goes on, it seems to get younger and younger." Unfortunately, at the present time, only our likenesses can stay young. But we can do plenty to slow down the processes of aging and developing illnesses (which could end the aging process as well).

Thirty percent of all U.S. adults age 65 and older have prediabetes, and another 30 percent have diabetes. More than 40 million people fall in that age range in the United States, which means that 12 million elderly have each condition. Because these people very often have other illnesses as well (like heart disease, kidney disease, decreased vision, and joint disease), they represent a very complicated group of patients with their own special needs.

In addition, the memory and thinking impairments that occur in the elderly can be made worse by prediabetes, diabetes, and obesity. This fact must be taken into consideration in any treatment plan. There is little value in a treatment plan if the patient is unable to follow it and has no one in his environment who can help.

Checking for memory and thinking disorders

A patient who can't take his medications or follow diet and exercise instructions is not going to be successful in reversing prediabetes or avoiding diabetes. For this reason, doctors must evaluate mental function in the elderly. Doing so may simply involve a standard examination that takes ten minutes to administer. One example is the St. Louis University Mental Status Examination, which asks 12 questions:

1. What day of the week is it? (1 point for the right answer)

2. What is the year? (1 point)

3. What state are we in? (1 point)

4. Remember these five objects. I will ask you what they are later: apple, pen, tie, house, car. (No points yet)

5. You have $100 and you go to the store and buy a dozen apples for $3 and a tricycle for $20.

    a. How much did you spend? (1 point)

    b. How much do you have left? (2 points)

6. Please name as many animals as you can in one minute. (No points for naming 0–5, 1 point for 5–10, 2 points for naming 10–15, and 3 points for more than 15)

7. What were the objects I asked you to remember? (1 point for each object named)

8. I am going to say a series of numbers and I would like you to give them to me backwards. For example, if I say 42, you would say 24.

    a. 87 (0 points)

    b. 649 (1 point)

    c. 8537 (1 point)

9. (Draw circle) This circle represents a clock face. Please put in the hour markers and the time at ten minutes to eleven o'clock. (2 points for hour markers labeled correctly, 2 points for correct time)

10. (Show a triangle, a square, and a rectangle) Please place an X in the triangle (1 point)

11. Which of the objects is the largest? (1 point)

12. I am going to tell you a story. Please listen carefully because afterward, I am going to ask some questions about it.

    Jill was a very successful stockbroker. She made a lot of money in the stock market. She then met Jack, a devastatingly handsome man. She married him and had three children. They lived in Chicago. She then stopped working and stayed at home to bring up her children. When they were teenagers, she went back to work. She and Jack lived happily ever after.

    a. What was the female's name? (2 points)

    b. When did she go back to work? (2 points)

    c. What work did she do? (2 points)

    d. What state did she live in? (2 points)

The exam is scored depending on whether the person is a high school graduate or not:

- ✔ **High school graduate:** Normal 27–30. Needs more evaluation 20–26. Dementia 1–19.

- ✔ **Less than high school graduate:** Normal 20–30. Needs more evaluation 14–19. Dementia 1–13.

The person can be reevaluated at intervals to assess whether his mental state is deteriorating or remaining steady. If this type of assessment reflects dementia, the patient will need help to take care of himself properly.

Considering kidney function

The diminishing function of one or both kidneys is partially responsible for blood glucose that's high. Blood flow to the kidney decreases by about 10 percent each decade after age 30 in a normal, healthy person. Circulation to the kidney is even less when high blood pressure or heart failure is present. Blood tests of kidney function may not reflect this decline because a key test measures the excretion of *creatinine*, a chemical that comes from muscle. With aging, muscle mass decreases along with the blood flow into the kidney, so less creatinine needs to be excreted and its level in the blood doesn't rise.

The main consequence of decreased blood flow to the kidney is the decreased ability of the kidney to get rid of salt, water, and glucose from the body. When the glucose rises to 180 mg/dl or higher, some is normally spilled into the urine. That process prevents the glucose from building up too high. The salt and water buildup causes the blood pressure to rise. Then the high blood pressure further decreases the kidney function. It's a vicious cycle.

Hormones coming from the adrenal gland, epinephrine and norepinephrine, are additional contributors to high glucose and blood pressure. Epinephrine raises blood pressure, heart rate, and blood glucose. Norepinephrine does the same thing. These hormones tend to be elevated in an elderly person's blood and don't fall as blood pressure rises.

Evaluating an elderly person's diet

If you don't live with the elderly person you're concerned about, you need to obtain a food history if at all possible because it represents such an important explanation for the development of prediabetes and diabetes. Ask the elderly person to write down *everything* she eats for three days. You may discover some of the following problems:

- ✔ Little fresh vegetable and fruit intake

- ✔ Little vitamin and mineral intake

- ✔ An excess of highly processed carbohydrates like cakes, candies, white rice, and white pasta

- ✔ Too much red meat

- ✔ Too much alcohol

You may want to steer her to a dietitian, who can develop a more balanced and lower calorie diet that's still enjoyable. Elderly people become less and less active with time, which is an important consideration in deciding how many calories someone should eat in a day.

Adding exercise to the program

Too often the elderly (especially the very elderly) do little or no exercise. This fact is very unfortunate because exercise not only prevents prediabetes in the elderly (just as it does in younger people) but also has a number of other benefits. For example, exercise

- ✔ Reduces the chance of a fall

- ✔ Adds strength and stamina

- ✔ Reduces the risk of high blood pressure

- ✔ Decreases the resting heart rate, making the heart more efficient

- ✔ Increases bone density to prevent fractures

- ✔ Relieves constipation

- ✔ Decreases stress

- ✔ Improves mental function and delays dementia

The number of elderly is growing significantly — by 2030, one in five Americans will be older than 65. For this reason, a growing number of professionals specialize in working with the "active aging" population. Go online and type "Specialist for Active Aging" in your Web browser to get an idea of what I'm talking about.

The elderly are often reluctant to exercise because they fear injury and pain in joints that already suffer from arthritis. They often don't realize that the opposite is true: By strengthening their muscles, they are able to function with less pain.

An elderly person starting an exercise program that will eventually be vigorous must consult with his doctor first. The doctor may conduct an exercise stress test. (Be aware that some doctors still believe exercise is dangerous for elderly people. If your doctor belongs to that group, find someone else to support your new lifestyle.)

Certain physical conditions may preclude doing aerobic exercise and resistance training:

- A recent heart attack
- Unstable chest pain
- Heart failure
- Uncontrolled high blood pressure
- Uncontrolled metabolic disease, like kidney or liver disease

Assuming these conditions don't apply and the doctor gives the green light to exercise, here are some guidelines for exercise in the elderly:

- Exercise sessions don't have to be 30 minutes long. Three 10-minute sessions are just as good.

- An elderly person (just like a younger person) should start slow and build up. He can walk just 10 minutes the first time, then 12, then 15, and so forth.

- Indoor training, especially on an exercise bike or an elliptical trainer, is just as good as outdoor exercise. Plus, these machines do not cause joint damage.

- The elderly should do strength and resistance training, as well as aerobic exercise. In Chapter 17 I show examples of resistance training exercises, which require a small investment in a few light weights. Muscle strength declines by 15 percent per decade after age 50 and 30 percent after age 70, but resistance training can result in 25 to 100 percent strength gains in older adults.

- Muscles grow stronger when they are overworked. The elderly should exercise to the point of muscle fatigue.

- Excellent ways of improving balance are standing on one foot and then the other, walking heel to toe, or doing Tai Chi.

- Someone who can't walk can still do exercises with her upper body, which will improve strength and stamina.

✔ Meeting with an exercise trainer once or twice can ensure that the person is doing the exercises properly.

✔ Walking in a pool is also an excellent way to exercise that minimizes the impact on joints while providing a satisfactory workout.

✔ The elderly should exercise at the maximal intensity at which they can still carry on a conversation. That intensity will increase over time.

Stopping the progression to diabetes

The elderly are often so burdened with other medications that they don't want to add another to prevent prediabetes from turning into diabetes. That's one reason that I always emphasize lifestyle change first. (The primary reason is that no pill is as effective as lifestyle change in reversing prediabetes and controlling diabetes.)

However, if a medication can be effective in reversing prediabetes and preventing diabetes, the benefit far outweighs the inconvenience. The medications used for the elderly to reverse prediabetes are the same as those used for younger persons (see Chapter 4 for details):

✔ Metformin, which has been shown to reduce the risk of diabetes in those with prediabetes by 31 percent.

✔ Actos, which actually reverses the insulin resistance at the root of prediabetes and may protect the insulin-secreting beta cells.

✔ Acarbose, which delays the absorption of carbohydrates in the intestine but leads to much gas and discomfort.

✔ Exenatide, which is injected twice daily and leads to weight loss while protecting the beta cells.

As I note elsewhere in the book, the U.S. Food and Drug Administration does not yet approve the use of these medications for prediabetes.

Bariatric surgery is another consideration for an elderly person. If the elderly person is in otherwise good health and can undergo surgery, this option should be considered. Treatments that would not have been tried in the past are being utilized more and more for older people as the technology becomes safer and the general health of the elderly improves.

Part IV
The Dangers of Moving toward Diabetes

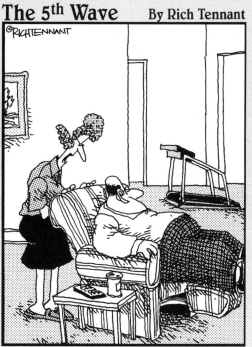

The 5th Wave   By Rich Tennant

"You know, anyone who wishes he had a remote control for his exercise equipment is missing the idea of exercise equipment."

In this part . . .

In this part, I present an extensive discussion of the possible consequences of moving from prediabetes to diabetes — both the short-term and the long-term consequences of diabetes left uncontrolled. One major concern is decreased sexual function, which affects both men and women. In addition, women have to deal with diabetes during pregnancy, which I fully explain here.

Chapter 12

Dealing with Short-Term Complications

*T*his and the next two chapters deal with the potential consequences if you let prediabetes become diabetes. Some complications, such as hypoglycemia, ketoacidosis, and hyperosmolar syndrome (all of which I describe in this chapter), can last for minutes or days and occur at any stage of diabetes. Others, which I discuss in the next two chapters, are long-term problems that take years of poorly controlled diabetes to develop.

The key thing is to get going on lowering your blood glucose now. Don't wait another day to begin to do the things that can prolong your life and increase its quality at the same time. You don't want to regret your life the way poor George Burns did. When a beautiful girl walked into his hotel room and said, "I'm sorry, I must be in the wrong room," he told her, "No, you're not in the wrong room. You are just 40 years too late."

You also don't want to be like the German poet Otto Hartleben. He was feeling very ill and consulted a doctor who, after a thorough examination, prescribed complete abstention from smoking and drinking. Hartleben picked up his coat and hat and started for the door. "That will be $30, Mr. Hartleben," said the doctor. "But I am not taking your advice," Hartleben replied, and left.

Watching Your Blood Glucose Drop: Hypoglycemia

Hypoglycemia means that your blood glucose level has fallen so low that you develop symptoms. Your brain doesn't work right. If you are a student, you have difficultly studying or taking tests. You can't perform acts that require coordination like driving a car or running complex machinery. You also have physical symptoms in addition to the mental symptoms.

A person with diabetes develops hypoglycemia not because of the disease itself but because of the medications she takes to control the disease. Other drugs, like alcohol and aspirin, can cause hypoglycemia as well, especially if the person doesn't eat enough food while consuming them.

 Three classes of medications that are commonly used for diabetes can cause hypoglycemia: insulin itself and the sulfonylurea drugs and meglitinides that act by getting the pancreas to release more insulin (see Chapter 18). Among the sulfonylurea drugs and meglitinides are the following:

- ✔ Glyburide, with brand names like Micronase, Diabeta, and Glynase
- ✔ Glipizide, with brands names like Glucotrol and Glucotrol XL
- ✔ Glimeperide, with the brand name Amaryl
- ✔ Repaglinide, with the brand name Prandin
- ✔ Nateglinide, with the brand name Starlix

Looking out for symptoms

The reason you develop symptoms is that both your brain and your muscles require glucose to function properly. Your muscles can turn to fat for energy when your blood glucose is low, but your brain requires glucose.

The level of blood glucose at which you develop hypoglycemic symptoms may be different for different people and even for the same person at different times. Most experts agree that a blood glucose of 60 mg/dl or less brings on signs and symptoms.

Symptoms fall into two major categories:

- ✔ *Adrenergic* symptoms refer to the symptoms that occur when your blood glucose falls rapidly. They are called adrenergic because in this situation, your body releases adrenaline to raise your blood glucose, and that action brings on many of the symptoms. The symptoms include:

- Anxiety
- Irritability
- Numbness of the lips, fingers, and/or toes
- Palpitations
- Rapid heartbeat
- Sensation of hunger
- Sweating
- Whiteness or pallor of the skin

✔ *Neuroglycopenic* symptoms result from not having enough glucose in your brain. They occur when your blood glucose falls more slowly, and they become more severe as your blood glucose falls lower. They include:

- Coma
- Confusion
- Convulsions
- Double vision or blurred vision
- Fatigue
- Feeling of warmth
- Headache
- Loss of concentration
- Poor color vision
- Slurred speech
- Trouble hearing

You can't think clearly if you are significantly hypoglycemic. You tend to make simple mistakes, and people may think you are drunk.

If you are taking any of the drugs I mention earlier in this section for treating diabetes, you should not skip meals or do heavy exercise (which uses up the glucose) without checking your blood glucose at the beginning and at intervals of every few hours.

Identifying the severity

Hypoglycemia can be classified into three levels of severity, approximately defined by the level of your blood glucose:

- ✔ Mild hypoglycemia is present at a blood glucose level of about 75 mg/dl. In this situation, the patient is aware of the problem and can treat himself. Mild hypoglycemia is often found when the patient routinely tests his blood glucose, and it accounts for the vast majority of cases.

- ✔ Moderate hypoglycemia occurs at a blood glucose level of about 65 mg/dl. The symptoms of rapid heartbeat and anxiety are prominent. The patient may be unaware that he is hypoglycemic and needs help from someone else.

- ✔ Severe hypoglycemia is found when the blood glucose is less than 55 mg/dl. The person can hardly function and must be treated by someone else to bring the glucose back up.

Treating hypoglycemia

Because most cases of hypoglycemia are mild, they are easily treated with a little sugar. You can buy glucose tablets over the counter that contain 15 grams of glucose in each. Two of them is usually enough to reverse hypoglycemia. Alternatively, drinking 4 ounces of apple juice or orange juice works well. The hypoglycemia should resolve in 20 minutes or less.

Moderate or severe hypoglycemia requires stronger measures. If the patient is having trouble staying conscious, an injection of *glucagon* (a hormone that helps regulate blood glucose) is required. You can find glucagon in several emergency kits available for people with diabetes, such as Glucagon Emergency Kit and GlucaGen Hypo Kit. The glucagon raises the patient's glucose so he regains consciousness and can take some food. Alternatively, the patient may be given an intravenous injection of glucose at high concentration. The trouble with that solution is that it is usually an overdose, and the patient's blood glucose goes very high.

Fighting Ketoacidosis

I introduce this dangerous complication of diabetes in Chapter 3, but I offer more detail here. Ketoacidosis occurs most often in patients with type 1 diabetes. Ketoacidosis is rare if you have type 2 diabetes, but it can occur, especially if you have another illness like an infection or a trauma that puts you under great stress.

The rate of developing ketoacidosis among the diabetic population seems to be increasing, but I don't have a clear explanation for that fact. Since 1999, the rate has increased from less than 3 percent per 10,000 people to more than 4 percent per 10,000 people. One explanation is the rising incidence of ketoacidosis in ethnic minority groups, especially African Americans and Hispanics. Although a precipitating cause (like infection or trauma) is usually present in these groups as well, ketoacidosis sometimes occurs without it.

Ketoacidosis is a severe complication, and some people die of this illness. The word *ketoacidosis* refers to the fact that your blood becomes very acidic as fat is broken down by your body for energy. *Keto* refers to the breakdown products of fat, which are called *ketone bodies.*

Looking out for symptoms

A number of symptoms can alert your loved ones that you have developed ketoacidosis. You may not be aware enough to recognize the problems yourself because you are so sick that your mental abilities are significantly reduced. The main signs and symptoms are

- ✔ **Nausea and vomiting:** These symptoms result from the acidic condition of your blood and the loss of many important body substances. You can't eat or drink, and you rapidly become dehydrated.

- ✔ **Rapid breathing:** Also called *Kussmaul breathing,* it occurs because your blood is so acidic that your body tries to get rid of the acid by blowing it out through your lungs. Your breath smells fruity from the acetone, one of the ketones.

- ✔ **Extreme tiredness and drowsiness:** You're tired because your blood is so thick with glucose that it's like syrup as it goes through your brain.

- ✔ **Weakness:** Even though the glucose in your blood is elevated, it can't get into your cells. As a result, your muscle tissue can't get its fuel, and you become extremely weak.

Ketoacidosis is too severe a complication to manage outside a hospital. You need to get to an emergency room where the doctor will find the following signs and test results:

- ✔ Acetone smell on your breath

- ✔ An acid condition of your blood, as determined by a blood test

- ✔ Deficiency of potassium, also shown by a blood test

- ✔ Dry skin and tongue resulting from dehydration

- ✔ Excessive levels of ketones in your blood and urine

- ✔ High blood glucose, usually over 300 mg/dl

Pinpointing causes

If you have diabetes, you can get ketoacidosis if you are on insulin and it is interrupted or if you suffer a severe infection or trauma. If you are dependent on insulin to control your blood glucose, ketoacidosis can occur within just a few hours of not having it.

There is a benign situation where your body uses fat and produces ketones: namely a strict diet. The big difference is that when you're dieting, your blood glucose remains low, your body does not become *acidotic* (meaning your blood plasma is acidic), and you are not sick.

Treating ketoacidosis

Treating ketoacidosis requires that your blood glucose be lowered into the normal range, that the acid condition of your blood be reversed, and that all the substances that are lost before treatment be replaced in your body, especially potassium and water.

The doctor will start you on an IV of salt water with some potassium if your blood potassium is low. She'll also start getting insulin into your system. After the insulin starts to flow, your body can use glucose for energy so that your high blood glucose begins to fall. Your body stops breaking down fat for energy, and the ketones derived from the breakdown of fat rapidly fall as well.

After your dehydration is improved with salt and water, you become much less nauseated and can start eating food and drinking liquids. Your normal mental function resumes, and you are able to administer your own insulin and test your own blood glucose. It takes about 24 to 36 hours to resume normal function.

Letting Your Blood Glucose Soar: Hyperosmolar Syndrome

The *hyperosmolar syndrome* is a condition in which the concentration of glucose in your blood rises to very high levels (600 mg/dl or more) as a result of a combination of dehydration, vomiting, and diarrhea. Unlike in ketoacidosis, your blood does not become very acidotic. The problem you experience is not due to a lack of insulin action; instead the loss of water in your system leads to very high concentrations of glucose.

The name *hyperosmolar syndrome* refers to the fact that concentrations of substances in your blood *(osmolar)* are very high *(hyper)*. As a result, your brain is bathed in syrupy blood, which may lead to coma.

The hyperosmolar syndrome is a medical emergency that is treated in the hospital. It usually occurs in people who are neglected in nursing facilities. No one notices that they are drinking very little and are vomiting and having diarrhea until their state of consciousness is very depressed.

Looking out for symptoms

Many of the symptoms of hyperosmolar syndrome are similar to those of ketoacidosis. But people with hyperosmolar syndrome do not have very acid blood and don't have the Kussmaul breathing that patients with ketoacidosis experience. Hyperosmolar syndrome develops over many days, while keto-acidosis may occur over several hours.

 If your blood glucose is measured regularly, hyperosmolar syndrome should not occur. But many patients who develop hyperosmolar syndrome are not even known to have diabetes and, therefore, don't have their glucose measured regularly.

These are the main signs and symptoms of hyperosmolar syndrome:

✔ Blood glucose of 600 mg/dl or higher

✔ Decreased mental awareness or coma

✔ Frequent urination

✔ High counts of blood potassium, sodium, red cells, and white cells due to the concentration of the blood

✔ Leg cramps

✔ Paralysis of the arms and legs

✔ Rapid pulse

✔ Sunken eyeballs

✔ Thirst

✔ Very low blood pressure

✔ Weakness

Pinpointing causes

As I note earlier, this condition tends to occur in people who are neglected, especially elderly people who live alone or are not monitored in nursing facilities. They become dehydrated, and no one notices.

Another problem is the gradual loss of kidney function with aging. As you get older, your kidneys do not leak glucose when your blood level is 180 mg/dl but at a higher level. So instead of the glucose in your blood being eliminated through the kidneys, it rises further. If you have lost fluids due to vomiting and/or diarrhea, your glucose concentration rises as your blood volume falls. The decreased blood volume also leads to decreased blood pressure, which further decreases the blood flow to the kidneys.

Infection, heart failure, failure to take insulin, and other factors found in elderly people may add more complications.

Treating hyperosmolar syndrome

Like ketoacidosis, this condition can't be treated at home. A doctor has to manage this condition, especially because most patients are elderly and have other diseases. The main treatment, which is replacement of the lost fluids, can easily be overdone, leading to fluid overload.

After diagnosis, the doctor accomplishes the following tasks very quickly:

- ✔ Looking for and treating a complicating factor such as an infection
- ✔ Lowering your blood glucose level
- ✔ Restoring large volumes of water to your body
- ✔ Restoring other substances that have been lost from your body, including sodium, potassium, and chloride

Little insulin is necessary in the treatment of hyperosmolar syndrome. The restoration of fluids brings your blood glucose down very nicely.

Identifying Other Annoyances of Diabetes

In addition to the three conditions I discuss in detail in this chapter, a number of minor problems are brought on by elevated blood glucose that can be managed fairly easily. But if your blood glucose is allowed to remain elevated, they will come back again. Among them are

- **Blurred vision:** This problem results from the alternating high and low blood glucose levels.

- **Frequent infections:** You'll also find that cuts and bruises heal poorly.

- **Frequent urination:** Your high blood glucose begins to spill out into your urine, drawing water out of your body so that your bladder is constantly full and you have to urinate often.

- **Itchy and dry skin:** Again, water being drawn out of your body into your bladder is the culprit.

- **Thirst:** The loss of water leads to dehydration and very significant thirst.

- **Tingling or numbness in your hands, legs, or feet:** This problem can also happen in prediabetes if that condition is allowed to go on for too long.

- **Vaginal infections in women:** As your tissues are bathed with higher levels of glucose than normal, they tend to develop yeast infections that go away with treatment but return rapidly if your blood glucose is not kept down. This problem can cause itching, an unpleasant odor, and discomfort during sex.

- **Weakness and fatigue:** Because glucose can't get into your cells as it should, the cells are starved for energy and you feel weak.

Chapter 13

Suffering Long-Term Consequences

*L*ong-term consequences of diabetes result from years of poor control of your blood glucose, as well as poor control of your blood pressure and blood cholesterol. It can take ten years or more for these complications to develop, so you have plenty of time to prevent them. However, after a time, the changes are fixed and become irreversible. That's why you want to prevent them as early as you can by not letting prediabetes turn into diabetes.

Some of the complications I discuss in this chapter — the eye disease and the nerve disease — have even been found in people with prediabetes, so you have even more reason to get your blood glucose under control as soon as possible.

The long-term consequences or complications of diabetes are divided into two groups: *microvascular* complications, which result from damage to the tiny blood vessels of the body; and *macrovascular* complications, which result from damage to the large blood vessels.

The microvascular complications include:

✔ Nephropathy: Damage to the kidneys with potential kidney failure

✔ Retinopathy: Damage to the eyes, including potential blindness

✔ Neuropathy: Damage to the nerves with potential loss of sensation, loss of muscular movement, and pain

The macrovascular complications include:

- ✔ Coronary artery disease and heart attacks due to the involvement of the coronary (heart) arteries
- ✔ Strokes due to the involvement of the cranial (head) arteries
- ✔ Peripheral vascular disease due to the involvement of the arteries to the legs and feet

You find out about all these issues and more in this chapter.

Grappling with Kidney Disease: Nephropathy

The function of your kidneys is to eliminate harmful chemicals and other materials formed in the course of normal metabolism. These substances are filtered through your kidneys and eliminated in your urine. Normal constituents of the body are sent back into your blood where they belong. The kidneys also regulate the salt and water content of your body. If your kidneys fail, you have two choices: have dialysis to artificially cleanse your body or have a kidney transplant to replace the damaged kidneys with a healthy kidney.

Fifty percent of patients undergoing long-term dialysis in the United States have had kidney failure due to diabetes. Thankfully, the incidence of new cases is declining because *nephropathy* (kidney disease) is being recognized early courtesy of the microalbumin test I describe later in this chapter.

What's happening to your kidneys?

Early in diabetes, your kidneys get larger as a result of the increased glucose and water that flow through them. They seem to be functioning even better than normal. However, changes are occurring in the tissues of the kidney that are the beginning of damage. The tissues are expanding and taking up space that should be open to the flow of fluids in the kidneys.

You normally have an excess of filtering tissue. In fact, you can get along on one kidney with little trouble. But if high blood glucose continues for about 15 years, you will have lost so much kidney function that substances that should be filtered out of your body will begin to back up and remain in your blood.

About 50 percent of the people whose blood glucose has been poorly controlled go on to develop nephropathy (kidney damage).

How high blood glucose leads to complications

Although doctors aren't certain about the causes of most long-term complications of diabetes, I mention the current theories about the causes of the complications as I explain each complication in this chapter. All long-term complications share some common characteristics:

✔ *Advanced glycated end products* (AGEs) are one of the substances that damage tissues. AGEs can damage your eyes, kidneys, nervous system, and other organs. You always have glucose in your blood, and some of that glucose attaches to other substances in your bloodstream to form *glycated* (glucose-attached) products. In this way, hemoglobin, which carries oxygen through your blood to cells and tissues throughout your body, attaches to glucose to form hemoglobin A1c. Albumin, a protein in blood, forms glycated albumin. Glucose can attach to red blood cells and white blood cells, as well as to other cells and molecules in the bloodstream. When these normal body substances attach to glucose, they no longer work normally.

When glucose attaches to other substances and cells, it alters their functions, usually in a negative fashion. For example, hemoglobin A1c holds on to oxygen more strongly than hemoglobin, so the cells that need oxygen don't get it as easily. Red blood cells that are glycated do not last as long in your blood circulation. Glycated white blood cells can't fight infection as well as unglycated white cells can.

Your body handles a certain level of glycated substances. But when your blood glucose is elevated for prolonged periods of time, the level of glycated cells and substances becomes excessive, and the complications I describe in this chapter result.

An interesting study in *Diabetes Care* in August 2005 showed that AGEs are present in higher amounts in patients with type 2 diabetes who develop peripheral arterial disease compared to those who don't develop it. The study suggests that AGEs play a role in large blood vessel disease as well as small blood vessel disease.

✔ The polyol pathway is another major source of damage to the body in diabetes. *Polyol pathway* refers to one direction, or pathway, that glucose can take as it is *metabolized* (broken down). For example, the common pathway is to form carbon dioxide and water as energy is produced. When you have a lot of glucose in your blood, an abnormal amount is metabolized to become a product called *sorbitol*. Sorbitol is a member of a class of substances called *polyols*. Sorbitol accumulates in many tissues where it can damage them in various ways:

Damage from swelling: Body water enters the cells to make the concentration of substances equal outside and inside, because sorbitol does not pass out of the cell. This causes damage and destruction of cells.

Damage from chemical reactions: During the production of sorbitol, other compounds are produced that chemically damage the cells and tissues.

Damage from autoantibodies: An article in 2005 in *Diabetes Care* showed that autoantibodies to autonomic nerves are present in patients with diabetes long before they suffer from autonomic neuropathy involving the heart and the peripheral autonomic nervous system. Autoimmunity may be yet another mechanism by which diabetes causes long-term complications.

(continued)

(continued)

> ✔ The protein kinase C pathway may be activated by elevated glucose levels. *Protein kinase C* is a substance that affects the way genes control the formation of many important proteins and other structures that are critical to health, including nerve cells. Abnormal formation of these structures can result in damage to nerves and other tissue.

> ✔ Abnormal amounts of fructose-6-phosphate may be generated by elevated glucose levels. Too much fructose-6-phosphate may lead to attachment of glucose to critical enzymes and growth factors so that these substances can't work properly, leading to damage in blood vessels.

Are there early signs of damage?

Fortunately, doctors do have a way to detect early on that kidney damage is occurring. A normal healthy kidney allows only tiny amounts of *albumin,* a protein, to escape into the urine. A kidney that is being damaged by diabetes allows significantly more albumin to escape. This amount can be measured either with a 24-hour urine specimen or with a random urine specimen (which is much less trouble). The test is called the *microalbuminuria test,* and it should be done annually for every patient with type 2 diabetes when diabetes starts and after five years of being diagnosed with type 1 diabetes.

If your level of microalbumin is elevated, you still have time to reverse the ongoing damage to your kidneys. But doing so requires that you take control of three key aspects of your health:

> ✔ You need to keep your blood glucose under tight control so that your hemoglobin A1c measurement (see Chapter 10) is under 7.

> ✔ You must lower your blood pressure to less than 130/80.

> ✔ You must reduce your total cholesterol to below 200 mg/dl.

I discuss these steps more in the next section.

Later, if your kidney disease worsens, the blood levels of certain chemicals may rise. These chemicals are the blood urea nitrogen (BUN) and serum creatinine. They are both normally eliminated by the filtering of the kidneys, and they back up into the blood when your kidneys are significantly damaged. Elevations in BUN and creatinine are signs of irreversible kidney damage and can be expected to worsen over time.

Kidney disease does not affect all people with diabetes equally. Certain ethnic groups — African Americans, Mexican Americans, and Native Americans — are more prone to develop kidney disease. It is also much more prevalent among people who have high blood pressure. High blood glucose seems to be the major cause, but only 50 percent of people with high blood glucose go on to develop nephropathy.

What are your treatment options?

Kidney failure is preventable. Two major studies, one for type 1 diabetes (the Diabetes Control and Complications Trial) and the other for type 2 diabetes (the United Kingdom Prospective Diabetes Study) have shown this fact conclusively. Here are the main steps you can take to reverse diabetic nephropathy or slow it down significantly:

- ✔ **Control your blood glucose:** The American Diabetes Association recommends keeping your hemoglobin A1c under 7 percent, while other experts suggest less than 6.5 percent. (I explain hemoglobin A1c and what these percentages mean in Chapter 10.) You experience the benefits not just at the time you control your blood glucose, but for years after.

- ✔ **Control your blood pressure:** If your doctor finds evidence of _microalbuminuria_ (too much of the protein albumin in your urine), you'll be started on a blood pressure drug from the class called _angiotensin-converting enzyme inhibitors,_ or ACE inhibitors. These drugs sometimes cause an uncomfortable cough, in which case a similar group of drugs called _angiotensin II receptor blockers_ can be used. See Chapter 18 for the details about these medications.

- ✔ **Control your blood fats:** You need to reduce your LDL or bad cholesterol and increase your HDL or good cholesterol. A class of drugs called _statins_ does this work very effectively, but other drugs are also effective (see Chapter 18).

- ✔ **Avoid additional kidney damage:** Urinary tract infections will hasten the damage to your kidneys so they must be treated. If you also have _neuropathy_ (nerve damage), which I discuss later in this chapter, you may not empty your bladder properly, and a urinary infection may result. You must actively manage this situation so you don't further damage your kidneys.

If you have kidney failure, you have two treatment options: dialysis or a kidney transplant. There are two forms of dialysis:

- ✔ **Hemodialysis:** A needle is placed in your artery, and your blood is pumped through a machine that filters out the toxic substances and returns the cleansed blood into your body. This process is usually done three times a week. Complications like low blood pressure and infection are possible.

> ✔ **Peritoneal dialysis:** A tube is placed in your abdominal cavity, which is called the *peritoneal cavity.* Fluid is dripped into your cavity, and it draws out the toxic wastes, which are then drained out with the fluid. This process is usually done at home but is not as efficient as hemodialysis, so it must be done daily. Sugar has to be used in the fluid, which can raise your blood glucose level unless insulin is also added. Peritoneal dialysis is also associated with infections where the tube enters the body cavity and within the peritoneal cavity.

Kidney transplantation is actually much easier than dialysis in the long run, but there are not a lot of available kidneys in the United States, so 80 percent of patients with kidney failure have dialysis and 20 percent have a transplant. The closer a kidney donor is to the recipient genetically, the lower the chance that the kidney will be rejected. But patients have to take anti-rejection drugs, which may complicate diabetic control. After a transplant operation, diabetic control is critical to protect the healthy kidney.

Coping with Eye Disease: Retinopathy

The second major site of damage done by uncontrolled diabetes is the eye. The damage is called *diabetic retinopathy* because the *retina,* the light-gathering tissue at the back of your eye, may be the most damaged.

People with diabetes also get *glaucoma,* which is high pressure damage to the eye, and *cataracts,* which involve the increasing opaqueness of the lens of the eye. However, these two conditions are not unique to diabetes. People with diabetes get both conditions earlier and more often than people without diabetes, but these conditions are very treatable.

An annual eye examination is a must for anyone with diabetes. Eye diseases that are diagnosed early are much more treatable than those that have already caused a lot of damage.

Ophthalmologists (eye doctors) divide retinopathy into two major forms:

> ✔ **Background retinopathy** is usually benign. The first signs are tiny dots on the back of your eye that are due to the ballooning of the capillaries to form aneurysms. Sometimes the aneurysms rupture and form retinal hemorrhages and *hard exudates,* which are scars from the hemorrhage. If these scars extend into the central light-gathering area of your retina called the *macula,* you may experience some loss of vision. If the capillaries leak into your macula, you may have *macular edema,* which can also cause a loss of vision.

Over time, the capillaries close, and the blood supply in the retina is diminished. Then you see cotton wool spots or *soft exudates,* which represent the destruction of your nerve fiber layer from lack of blood supply. About half the time this condition goes on to become the more serious proliferative retinopathy.

✔ **Proliferative retinopathy** results in vision loss if not treated. Because the blood supply to your retina is reduced, new blood vessels form, which can hemorrhage in front of your retina and block your vision. The hemorrhage forms a clot and retracts. It can pull your retina forward and cause retinal detachment and complete loss of vision.

Fortunately, excellent treatment is available for proliferative retinopathy. Laser treatment is used to create burns that scar your retina and prevent it from detaching. This procedure works 95 percent of the time. If your retina has already detached, a surgical procedure called *vitrectomy* may be used to cut the attachments to your retina and allow it to fall back into place. Vitrectomy works 90 percent of the time.

Facing Nerve Disease: Neuropathy

Your nervous system is the third major organ system that is attacked by poorly controlled diabetes. *Neuropathy* (nerve disease) may affect 60 percent of people with diabetes. The incidence increases with the increasing duration of diabetes. Most people with neuropathy have long had poorly controlled diabetes, smoke cigarettes, drink alcohol excessively, and are older than 40. However, as young people are getting diabetes more frequently, we will see neuropathy in younger and younger patients.

Diagnosing neuropathy

Neuropathy is usually diagnosed by doing a test with a filament that looks like a hair. The filament that is used usually bends with 10 grams of force. People who can feel that filament should be able to feel any sensation that may damage their feet, such as a nail in a shoe or a stone.

Other ways of testing the nerves include using a tuning fork to detect the loss of vibration sense and the use of hot or cold items to detect the loss of temperature sensation. Obviously, not being able to detect something that is excessively hot can result in a burn.

Recognizing symptoms

Depending upon which nerves are affected, the symptoms of neuropathy fall into the following categories:

- Disorders of loss of sensation
- Disorders of loss of motor nerves
- Disorders of loss of *autonomic* nerves, the nerves that control muscles automatically (like the heart, lungs, and intestines)
- Entrapment neuropathies, which are disorders resulting from the swelling of nerves as they pass through bones.

I discuss each group of disorders in turn.

Disorders of sensation

These are the most common conditions that occur when neuropathy is present. They break down into two categories: *diffuse neuropathies,* where many nerves are involved; and *focal neuropathies,* where only one or a few nerves are affected.

The various kinds of diffuse neuropathies include the following:

- **Distal polyneuropathy:** This condition, involving the hands and/or feet, is the most common form of neuropathy. When you have this condition, you lose the sensation of light touch, and you often experience tingling and burning, a loss of balance, and a worsening of the symptoms at night. You may also have a minimal loss of strength. Damage to your feet may occur because you simply don't feel it happening. Infection may set in, which could even lead to amputation.

- **Diabetic amyotrophy:** This condition involves pain and loss of muscle strength in the muscles of your upper leg so you can't straighten your knee. This condition usually improves after several months.

- **Radiculopathy:** This pain all along the length of a nerve suggests that the root of the nerve is damaged. It can be very severe, but it resolves in 6 to 24 months.

Focal neuropathies can affect any nerve so that small areas of loss of sensation or pain may occur anywhere in the body.

Disorders of movement

Just about any single nerve can suddenly be affected by this type of disorder, and the muscle that the nerve is attached to is then unable to move. The suddenness suggests that this condition involves the sudden closing of a blood vessel that supplies that nerve. The symptoms depend on which nerve is affected. For example, if a nerve to your eye muscle is affected, you won't be able to turn the eye toward the side the muscle is on. This disorder resolves itself in time.

Disorders of autonomic nerves

The *autonomic* nerves control the automatic movements in your body: your heart muscles, your diaphragm that controls breathing, the movement of your intestinal muscles to push food along, your bladder muscles, and so forth.

Depending upon the nerve that is affected, this type of disorder may lead to one of the following conditions:

- **Bladder abnormalities:** They begin with the loss of the sensation of bladder fullness. When this happens, you may get urinary tract infections because your bladder is not fully emptied. This condition can be diagnosed by observing how much urine is left in your bladder after you have tried to empty it. If you have this problem, you must urinate regularly regardless of whether you feel the need to do so.

- **Gallbladder disease:** The gallbladder doesn't empty the way it usually does each time you eat, especially after a fatty meal. Gallstones may form.

- **Heart disease:** The nerves to your heart are lost, and you may become light-headed when you stand. You may also experience a fast fixed heart rate.

- **Large intestinal problems:** The results may be diabetic diarrhea, the accidental loss of bowel contents, and an abnormal growth of bacteria.

- **Sexual dysfunction:** I discuss this topic in detail in Chapter 14.

- **Stomach problems:** Your body may fail to empty the complete contents of your stomach — a condition called *gastroparesis.* When this happens, your diabetes can be difficult to control because the timing of the absorption of food does not correlate with the timing of the action of the medication you take to lower the glucose.

- **Sweating problems:** These occur especially in the feet. Your body compensates by sweating more in your upper body (your face and trunk). Eating cheese can provoke heavy sweating because a substance in cheese causes the widening of blood vessels under the skin.

Entrapment neuropathies

These conditions occur when various nerves swell and are trapped and squeezed as they pass through bony areas. The entrapment neuropathy that most people know about is *carpal tunnel syndrome,* where a nerve is trapped at the wrist, resulting in decreased sensation and weakness of the hand.

The entrapment neuropathies include the following:

- **Carpal tunnel syndrome:** With this condition, you experience reduced sensation in your fingers and weakness when you touch your thumb to your fifth finger. The *median nerve* (which runs down your arm and forearm) is trapped at your wrist.

- **Ulnar nerve entrapment:** You experience reduced sensation in part of your fourth finger and your entire fifth finger. Your hand loses sensation between your fifth finger and wrist. The ulnar nerve is trapped at the elbow.

- **Radial nerve entrapment:** You lose sensation in the back of your hand and experience "wrist drop" from the loss of the muscles that straighten up your wrist. The radial nerve is trapped at the elbow.

- **Common peroneal nerve entrapment:** You lose sensation in the side of your leg and the top of your foot, and you experience "foot drop" from weakness of the muscles that pull up your foot. The common peroneal nerve is trapped as it passes the head of the fibula.

- **Tarsal tunnel syndrome:** You lose sensation on both sides of your foot and experience a wasting of the foot muscles, resulting in decreased toe movement. This condition results from the trapping of the tibial nerve between two of the small foot bones.

- **Lateral femoral cutaneous nerve entrapment:** You lose sensation on the outside of your thigh but experience no muscle weakness. It results from the trapping of that nerve at the groin.

The treatment for entrapment neuropathies consists of rest, splints, drugs to promote water loss and reduce swelling, injections of steroids, and surgery if needed. These conditions should not be confused with the focal neuropathies I discuss earlier in this chapter.

Diabetic neuropathy can be a real pain because so many potential conditions exist. Wouldn't it be a whole lot easier and better to avoid the whole thing by turning your prediabetes into normal glucose metabolism with some good lifestyle changes?

Putting Your Heart at Risk

Deaths due to coronary artery disease and heart attacks have been declining over the last 30 years, but with the huge increase in cases of type 2 diabetes, this trend may be about to reverse. Heart disease may occur much earlier in life because young patients are getting type 2 diabetes at such a rapid rate.

Following are some of the factors that promote coronary artery disease in diabetes:

✔ Abnormal blood fats — especially reduced HDL (good) cholesterol and increased triglyceride. These abnormal fats may not improve when your blood glucose is controlled and may be present in prediabetes as well as diabetes.

✔ Central obesity, which I discuss in Chapter 9. This phrase refers to carrying much of your excess weight around your middle.

✔ High blood pressure.

✔ The increased production of insulin due to insulin resistance.

✔ Obesity.

People with diabetes have more extensive coronary artery disease than people without diabetes. The risk of death from a heart attack is greater in people with diabetes. Half the people who have diabetes will die from a heart attack.

While a non-diabetic dies only 15 percent of the time from a heart attack, a person with diabetes dies 40 percent of the time. And the complication rate is much greater for the person with diabetes. The death rate at five years after the heart attack is 80 percent for the person with diabetes and only 25 percent for the person without diabetes.

Trust me: Your heart does not want you to have diabetes.

Realizing the role of the metabolic syndrome

The metabolic syndrome, which I discuss in detail in Chapter 9, results from insulin resistance and greatly contributes to the dangers of coronary artery disease in people with diabetes. Insulin resistance is associated with three times the incidence of coronary artery disease compared to people with normal insulin sensitivity. Insulin resistance leads to:

✔ Blood fat abnormalities that promote blood vessel disease

✔ An increase in C-reactive protein, which indicates inflammation is playing a role

✔ High blood pressure from increased insulin

✔ Increased blood clot formation

✔ Increased *visceral* fat (the bad fat that hangs around your middle)

✔ Microalbuminuria, which points to both kidney disease and coronary artery disease

All these changes promote coronary artery disease.

Feeling the effects of nerve disease

In the previous section, I discuss many of the ways your body may be affected by a loss of nerve control. Your heart is one of the organs that may be affected, and the result is a condition called *cardiac autonomic neuropathy*.

Your doctor can make this diagnosis by measuring your pulse and blood pressure:

✔ Your resting heart rate may be abnormally high.

✔ Your standing blood pressure may fall abnormally low (a decrease of 20 mm of mercury) compared to your sitting blood pressure.

✔ The variation in your heart rate with breathing may be too low. The variation should be greater than 10 between inspiration and expiration, but if you have nerve disease, your heart rate does not vary as much.

People with cardiac autonomic neuropathy may have a decreased chance of survival even if they don't have coronary artery disease.

Dealing with an enlarged heart

If you have *cardiomyopathy,* you have an enlarged heart and scarring of the heart muscle even where there is little or no coronary artery disease. The heart is failing and can't pump enough blood. If you also have high blood pressure, your heart will fail even sooner.

The best treatment is a combination of lowering your blood glucose and lowering your blood pressure.

Avoiding a Stroke

Diabetes can cause *cerebrovascular disease:* disease of the blood vessels to the *cerebrum,* or brain.

Smoking and diabetes

As you well know, smoking has a number of ill effects on people without diabetes, but the effects are even worse in people with diabetes. Among other things, smoking:

✔ Reduces blood flow in arteries and blocks increased flow when it is needed

✔ Increases pain in the legs in people with peripheral vascular disease and in the heart in people with coronary artery disease

✔ Increases *atheromatous plaques,* the changes in arteries in the heart and other areas (like the brain and the legs) that precede closing of the blood vessels

✔ Increases the clustering of *platelets,* the blood elements that form a plug or clot that blocks the artery

✔ Increases blood pressure, which also worsens atheromatous plaques

These problems don't even take into account the effects of smoking on the lungs, the bladder, and the rest of the body. Whatever your cholesterol level, smoking has the effect of adding 100 mg/dl to that level. So if your measurement is 250 mg/dl, your effective cholesterol is 350 mg/dl.

The blood supply to part of your brain may be blocked temporarily due to the spasm of arteries or a clot that is quickly broken up in an artery. This situation is called a *transient ischemic attack* (TIA). A TIA may cause temporary symptoms such as:

✔ Slurring of speech

✔ Weakness on one side of your body

✔ Numbness on one side of your body

The symptoms may disappear within minutes and return sometime later. Or a full stroke may occur later with permanent loss of function.

Just as people with diabetes experience more extensive disease in the blood vessels to the heart (compared with people who don't have diabetes), they also experience more extensive damage in blood vessels to the brain. Many small vessels may be blocked, and the result can be the gradual loss of intellectual function that appears like Alzheimer's disease.

The effects of a stroke may be reversed if you are treated with clot-busting drugs early enough — within three hours of developing symptoms. If you ever experience the symptoms I list earlier in this section, get to an emergency room as soon as you can.

You can minimize your risk of a stroke by acting now to do the following:

- ✔ Lower your blood glucose
- ✔ Lower your blood pressure
- ✔ Lower your cholesterol
- ✔ Reduce your weight
- ✔ Stop smoking

Fighting Peripheral Vascular Disease

Peripheral vascular disease (PVD) refers to damage of the blood vessels other than the coronary (heart) vessels and the cerebral (brain) vessels. It begins earlier and proceeds more rapidly in someone with diabetes than in someone who doesn't have diabetes. The term mostly refers to the disease of major arteries in the legs.

Normally, you can feel the pulses of blood vessels on top of your foot and along the sides of your foot. But if you have diabetes and have had ten or more years of poor control of your blood pressure, blood glucose, and cholesterol, you have about a one-third chance of no longer having pulses that can be felt.

The major symptoms of PVD depend on which arteries are most affected. Usually you experience pain in your calves, thighs, or buttocks that starts with walking and subsides with rest. That's because walking increases the need for blood in your tissues. The blockage prevents the artery from increasing the blood flow.

If the pain is present even at rest, it suggests you have very substantial blockage. Then your doctor will perform an angiogram of the affected blood vessels. If your doctor confirms the blockage, he'll recommend surgery to open the blood vessel. Sometimes in diabetes the vascular damage is so extensive that surgery can't be done; amputation may be the only course.

An excellent screening test for PVD is called the *ankle-brachial index* (ABI). The systolic blood pressure in your ankle is measured, along with the systolic blood pressure in your arm. The ankle pressure is divided by the arm pressure. Normally, the result should be .95 or more. A value of .75 or less suggests significant peripheral vascular disease.

Amputating Due to Diabetic Foot Disease

Diabetic foot disease is completely avoidable. Yet thousands of amputations are performed every year as a result of this condition. That's because patients fail to do certain routine things like visually inspecting their feet for lesions every day, testing their feet for sensation, and applying moisturizers and lubricants to protect their feet.

When you have diabetic foot disease, pressure on your feet results in ulcers that can lead to the need for amputation. You can do a number of things to prevent this sequence from occurring:

- Change your shoes every five hours.
- Don't use a heating pad on your feet.
- If you have new shoes, change them every two hours at first.
- Inspect your feet daily. Use a mirror to see every part.
- Never walk barefoot.
- Shake out your shoes before you put them on.
- Stop smoking. The combination of smoking and diabetes is a major cause of amputations.

Treatment of a diabetic ulcer is done by taking pressure off the involved foot and elevating it. Sometimes a plaster cast is applied to keep the pressure off the ulcer. Any dead tissue is carefully removed, and any infection is treated with antibiotics. A product called Regranex Gel may also be applied to the cleaned ulcer daily, which promotes the regrowth of healthy tissue. It may take three to four months for the ulcer to fully heal.

See a podiatrist at the first sign of a foot lesion associated with diabetes. This step may be the most important thing you can do to avoid an amputation.

Suffering with Diabetic Skin Disease

Diabetes can affect every part of the body. As proof, consider that a number of skin diseases are associated with diabetes. These include:

- *Acanthosis nigricans,* a velvety-feeling increase in pigmentation on the neck, the armpits, and other sites. This condition is benign and needs no treatment but is often seen in children with type 2 diabetes.

- ✔ *Alopecia,* or hair loss. usually seen in type 1 diabetes.
- ✔ Bruises from cutting your skin with the insulin needle.
- ✔ Diabetic thick skin, which occurs after more than ten years of diabetes.
- ✔ Dry skin from diabetic neuropathy.
- ✔ Fungal infections under the nails or between the toes from the increased glucose and moisture in diabetes.
- ✔ *Insulin hypertrophy,* which is an accumulation of fat tissue where insulin is injected.
- ✔ *Insulin lipoatrophy,* which is a loss of fat tissue where insulin is injected.
- ✔ *Necrobiosis lipoidica,* or reddish-brown skin patches on the shins and ankles, especially in females. They are more unsightly than dangerous. They can be injected with steroids and become depressed and brown.
- ✔ *Vitiligo,* a loss of skin pigmentation, which is an autoimmune disease that accompanies type 1 diabetes.
- ✔ *Xanthelasma,* which presents as yellow, flat areas on the eyelids.

This list is long, but fortunately none of these conditions is dangerous — only unsightly.

Experiencing Diabetic Gum Disease

When you have diabetes, the higher-than-normal concentration of glucose in your mouth promotes gum disease. Food mixes with saliva and germs to form plaques on your gums. You need to brush your teeth twice a day and floss daily to prevent these plaques from hardening into tartar, which is removed only with great effort by your dentist.

If your gums become brittle and bleed easily, you have *gingivitis.* Then you have pain and bad breath. Your gums can become so damaged that they are unable to support your teeth.

The keys to avoiding diabetic gum disease are controlling your blood glucose, brushing and flossing your teeth daily, and visiting your dentist for routine cleaning twice a year.

Interestingly, people with diabetes do not have more cavities than people who don't have diabetes.

Chapter 14

Risking Your Sexual Health: Sexual Function and Pregnancy

. . . .

In This Chapter

▶ Creating sexual problems for women

▶ Recognizing risks of diabetes during pregnancy

▶ Impairing a man's sexual performance

. . . .

Sexual function is a key part of our lives. Not only does it allow the species to continue and provide a wonderful source of pleasure, but it's also the way that many matchmaking services on the Internet earn their money. (Ah, capitalism!)

Diabetes can have a profound effect on sexual function in both women and men, in both the short term and long term. In this chapter, I tell you about these entirely avoidable complications and give you another reason, I hope, not to allow your prediabetes to progress to diabetes.

Considering How Diabetes Affects Women's Sexual Function

Women can develop a variety of sexual problems when they have high blood glucose levels and when they suffer tissue damage after having diabetes for a long time. As many as 35 percent of women with diabetes suffer from sexual dysfunction.

Here are some of the short-term sexual problems caused by diabetes:

✔ A feeling of lack of attractiveness because type 2 diabetes is usually associated with obesity

✔ A feeling of lack of sexual interest or desire

- ✔ Dry mouth and dry vagina as a result of high blood glucose levels

- ✔ Irregular menstrual function when your blood glucose is out of control

- ✔ A reduction in estrogen, which leads to thinning and dryness of the vagina

- ✔ Yeast infections of the vagina that make intercourse unpleasant

All these problems can be exacerbated if you don't feel comfortable speaking to your doctor or partner about them.

Here are some of the long-term sexual problems due to damage to nerves and blood vessels:

- ✔ Decreased blood flow (due to blood vessel disease associated with diabetes), which causes decreased vaginal lubrication

- ✔ Loss of bladder control due to nerve disease in your bladder (see Chapter 13)

- ✔ Loss of skin sensation around the vaginal area and on the clitoris because of nerve disease

- ✔ Reduced lubrication (making entry of the penis more difficult and decreasing your pleasurable sensation), also the result of nerve disease

Women can greatly improve their lubrication with over-the-counter lubricants like K-Y jelly and In Pursuit of Passion. Petroleum-based lubricants are not recommended because they may contribute to bacterial infections.

If lack of desire is the issue, reading erotic books or viewing erotic videotapes may help.

Working with a therapist may help some of the psychological issues, especially depression. However, antidepressant medication may cause vaginal dryness and the inability to have an orgasm. Be sure to weigh the pros and cons of antidepressants with your physician. Therapy with your partner may also help to enhance your sexual pleasure.

The best treatment for all these problems is preventative. Keeping your blood glucose under control, keeping your blood pressure normal, and maintaining a normal cholesterol level will permit you to enjoy sex as it should be enjoyed.

Focusing on Pregnancy

When a woman is pregnant, she tends to be totally cooperative with her doctor. She is caring not just for herself but for her unborn baby, and she will gladly do anything a doctor asks to deliver a healthy child.

During pregnancy, as a result of the stresses and the increased levels of hormones that are produced, prediabetes can turn into diabetes. Diabetes that develops during a pregnancy is called *gestational diabetes.* It occurs in up to 10 percent of all pregnancies, and the numbers are rising.

Having diabetes during pregnancy can be very complicated. That's why centers devoted to managing diabetic pregnancies have sprung up around the country. If your prediabetes turns into diabetes during your pregnancy, you may consider taking advantage of the expertise to be found there.

Even though going through a pregnancy with diabetes can be tough, it is possible to produce a totally healthy mother and child at delivery. All the tools that are needed are available. The challenge is using them properly.

And even better is avoiding letting your prediabetes turn into diabetes while you're pregnant. In this section, I offer you the information you need to make that happen.

Diagnosing gestational diabetes

Because diabetes is a silent disease, pregnant women must be screened in order to discover it.

Who should be screened?

The incidence of gestational diabetes is high: One in ten pregnant women develops it. But screening all pregnant women is not cost-effective. Therefore, if you meet the following criteria, you likely will *not* be screened (because you likely will not develop gestational diabetes):

✔ You are younger than 25.

✔ You had a normal weight before the pregnancy.

✔ You are not a member of an ethnic group with a high incidence of type 2 diabetes, such as Latinos, African Americans, Native Americans, and Pacific Islanders.

✔ You have no family history of diabetes (meaning diabetes in your parents, siblings, or other children).

✔ You have no previous history of intolerance to glucose.

✔ You have no previous history of a poor outcome of a birth or having a large baby.

Factors that make screening mandatory include:

✔ Previous delivery of a large baby

✔ Obesity

✔ Glucose in your urine

✔ A close family member with diabetes

How screening is done

Initial screening for gestational diabetes is usually done between the 24th and 28th weeks of pregnancy. It's done earlier if you've had a previous pregnancy with gestational diabetes. You don't have to do any preparation for the screening. You're simply given 50 grams of glucose to drink, and your blood glucose is measured an hour later. Any value of more than 140 mg/dl is considered abnormal and is followed by a more definitive test. The definitive test is done in the following way:

✔ You prepare by eating at least 150 grams of carbohydrate daily for three days and fasting for eight hours before the test.

✔ You drink 100 grams of glucose.

✔ Your blood glucose is measured before you drink the glucose and at one hour, two hours, and three hours after drinking the glucose.

✔ A diagnosis of gestational diabetes is made if two or more of your blood glucose samples exceed the levels shown in Table 14-1.

Table 14-1	Excessive Glucose Levels That Signal Gestational Diabetes		
Before	*1 Hour*	*2 Hours*	*3 Hours*
95 mg/dl (5.3 mmol/L)	180mg/dl (10.0 mmol/L)	155 mg/dl (8.6 mmol/L)	140 mg/dl (7.8 mmol/L)

Understanding the consequences to mother and baby

If your blood glucose is not controlled, you may have trouble even conceiving a baby. You may also experience more frequent miscarriages than someone whose blood glucose is normal. And if you have uncontrolled diabetes before your baby is conceived, you risk that your baby will develop congenital malformations of the heart, central nervous system, skeleton, kidneys, and intestines.

Developing gestational diabetes at week 24 or after brings on the possibility of other risks for both the mother and the baby. The baby may be large because of fat storage in the shoulders, chest, abdomen, arms, and legs. Large babies are often delivered early to avoid birth trauma for the baby and the mother, or they are delivered by caesarean section. A baby is considered to be large if he weighs more than 9 pounds at birth.

Keep in mind that most large babies are not due to diabetes. However, large babies born to mothers without diabetes have proportional growth of their shoulders and heads, which means that delivery is usually not as complicated.

Treating diabetes during pregnancy

With gestational diabetes, it's important that you maintain a stricter level of blood glucose control than when you are not pregnant. The fetus removes glucose from your blood, so your blood glucose is lower than usual. Your body turns to fat for energy much earlier in a pregnancy so you produce the breakdown products of fat, *ketones,* much earlier. This condition is called *accelerated starvation.* Too many ketones are bad for the fetus.

Gaining the right amount of weight

In 2009, the Institute of Medicine published new guidelines for weight gain during pregnancy. Previous guidelines 20 years ago emphasized the needs of the baby, but these new guidelines recognize the needs of the mother as well.

Here are the recommended guidelines for pregnancy weight gain, which are categorized according to your prepregnancy body mass index (BMI), which I explain in detail in Chapter 6:

- ✔ If you are underweight (have a BMI less than 18.5), your pregnancy gain should be 28 to 40 pounds.

- ✔ If you are normal weight (have a BMI of 18.5 to 24.9), your pregnancy gain should be 25 to 35 pounds.

- ✔ If you are overweight (have a BMI of 25.0 to 29.9), your pregnancy gain should be 15 to 25 pounds.

- ✔ If you are obese (have a BMI more than 29.9), your pregnancy gain should be 11 to 20 pounds.

If you have prediabetes or diabetes, you should meet with a dietitian to work out a diet that provides enough carbohydrates and sufficient weight gain for the pregnancy. Taking a good multivitamin and mineral preparation will also help keep your pregnancy a healthy one.

Monitoring your glucose and ketones

If you have gestational diabetes, it's critically important to maintain normal blood glucose levels. The recommended levels are shown in Table 14-2.

Table 14-2	Optimum Levels of Blood Glucose	
Fasting and Premeal	*1 Hour after Eating*	*2 Hours after Eating*
Less than 90 mg/dl (5 mmol/L)	Less than 120 mg/dl (6.7 mmol/L)	Less than 120 mg/dl (6.7 mmol/L)

If your blood glucose is not kept at the levels shown in Table 14-2, you need to be on insulin shots. Someone who refuses to take shots can use *glyburide*, a drug that stimulates increased insulin but does not pass through the placenta, although this use is not approved by the Food and Drug Administration. If you do take insulin, you stop taking it at the time of delivery.

You should also be checking for ketones in your urine by placing a test strip into your stream of urine. If the test strip is positive, it means you are breaking down fat for energy because you are not taking in enough carbohydrates.

Testing for fetal defects

If you have gestational diabetes, several tests are done to ensure that your pregnancy is going well and the baby is doing fine. The key tests are

- ✔ **Serum alpha-fetoprotein:** This blood test is done 15 weeks into the pregnancy to determine whether certain congenital malformations are present.

- ✔ **Ultrasound:** This study bounces sound off the fetus to show any malformations. It does not hurt the growing fetus.

- ✔ **Non-stress test:** In this study, a device is placed over the abdomen to listen to the heartbeat of the fetus. When the fetus moves, the heart rate normally goes up by 15 to 20 beats per minute, and this normally happens at least three times in a 20-minute period of listening.

Delivering the baby

Your baby must be given the chance for maximum development in your uterus before delivery. Delivery usually takes place at 39 weeks. If you don't go into labor spontaneously, your obstetrician will induce labor. If necessary, you'll be given insulin to keep your blood glucose between 70 and 120 mg/dl. Only short-acting insulin is used because you don't want insulin in your circulation when it's no longer needed.

Monitoring the mother after delivery

Most times, gestational diabetes goes away after the mother is no longer exposed to the glucose-raising hormones of pregnancy. However, a woman who develops gestational diabetes is at increased risk to develop type 2 diabetes later in life. If you have a fasting blood glucose test greater than 130 mg/dl during pregnancy, you have a 75 to 90 percent chance of later developing type 2 diabetes. It's critical to lose all your pregnancy weight and begin an exercise program as soon as possible.

Women who have gestational diabetes are tested for glucose tolerance between 6 and 12 weeks after the pregnancy and annually thereafter if diabetes is not found.

If you have gestational diabetes, certain factors that are out of your control will predispose you to getting type 2 diabetes later in life:

- ✔ **Ethnicity:** If you are Mexican American, Native American, Asian American, or African American, your risk is higher.
- ✔ **A family history of diabetes:** Having a family member with diabetes means your risk is higher.
- ✔ **Number of pregnancies:** The more pregnancies you've had, the greater your risk.
- ✔ **Loss of blood glucose control during pregnancy:** The more severe the loss of control, the greater your risk.
- ✔ **Weight prior to pregnancy:** The higher this number, the greater the risk.

But other factors that can contribute to type 2 diabetes are very much in your control:

- ✔ Dietary fat
- ✔ Future pregnancies
- ✔ Future weight gain
- ✔ Physical activity
- ✔ Smoking and certain drugs

Monitoring the baby after delivery

Your baby may develop a number of problems if your blood glucose was not controlled during pregnancy. The most important problems include:

- **Hyperbilirubinemia:** Too many blood cells break down, causing the baby's skin to turn yellow.

- **Hypoglycemia:** The baby has been exposed to high glucose in the uterus and makes a lot of insulin. Suddenly, the high glucose is cut off at birth. The large amount of insulin still present may cause a severe drop in blood glucose in the baby. The baby may be sweaty, appear nervous, or have a seizure. This condition usually subsides by six hours after delivery.

- **Low calcium:** This problem is due to prematurity.

- **Low magnesium:** This problem is also due to prematurity.

- **Respiratory distress syndrome:** The baby's breathing tubes are not fully mature, and breathing may be difficult.

All these conditions are very treatable but — even better — are avoidable if your blood glucose is kept under control.

Impacting Men's Sexual Performance

More than 50 percent of men with diabetes have difficulty with their sexual function. The difficulty is called *erectile dysfunction* (ED), which means an inability to have or sustain an erection sufficient for intercourse. ED develops 10 to 15 years earlier in men with diabetes than in men who don't have it. After age 70, more than 95 percent of men with diabetes have ED.

Explaining erectile dysfunction

Other causes for ED must be ruled out before blaming diabetes. These include:

- Hormonal abnormalities like too little testosterone

- Medications like blood pressure pills and antidepressants

- Poor blood supply to the penis from peripheral vascular disease

- *Psychogenic impotence,* where the loss of erectile function is limited to a certain partner or partners

- Trauma to the penis

A successful erection requires that the nerves to the penis work properly. Diabetes can damage these nerves so that erections can't take place. Certain nerves cause muscles to relax so that more blood flows into the penis. Other muscles contract under the influence of nerves so that semen is propelled through the penis while the bladder is shut off for ejaculation to take place.

A number of factors determine when ED will begin, especially the degree of control of your blood glucose, the duration of diabetes, and your use of alcohol or other drugs that interfere with erections.

Treating erectile dysfunction

A man who has erectile dysfunction, whether he has diabetes or not, has all kinds of possibilities for treatment. Most treatment begins with drugs, goes on to external devices that create an erection, and continues to implantable devices that produce an erection.

Drug treatment

The availability of Viagra, the brand name for the drug sildenafil, has revolutionized the treatment of ED. This drug and two others, Levitra (the brand name for vardenafil) and Cialis (the brand name for tadalafil), all work in the same way to produce erections. They are successful in 70 percent of patients.

As I note earlier, certain muscles need to relax to allow a lot of blood to flow into the penis. This process takes place when a nerve releases a chemical that is taken up by the muscle to cause relaxation. A second chemical then breaks down the first so increased blood flow stops. These three drugs all work by blocking the action of that second chemical. So Viagra and the others require some stimulation to get the first chemical flowing. Then they can work to stop the second chemical. The stimulation may be tactile (touch), visual, oral, auditory, or whatever a man finds exciting.

The drugs have some side effects like facial flushing, headaches, and indigestion, but these decline as drug use continues. Viagra and Levitra work in a similar way. They are taken an hour before sexual intercourse. The dose of Viagra is 50 mg and Levitra 10 mg, but many men with diabetes require twice that dose. The pills' effects last for four hours. The dose of Cialis is 20 mg (40 mg for diabetic men), and its action begins in 20 minutes and lasts 36 hours.

Certain drugs can be injected directly into the blood vessels of the penis to relax them and allow more blood flow. These include papaverine, phentolamine, and Alprostadil. They are injected 30 minutes prior to intercourse.

A suppository form of Alprostadil is also available, which is injected into the *urethra,* the tube through which urine and semen pass. This preparation, called MUSE, is used every 12 hours and does not require stimulation.

External devices

Vacuum devices can be placed over the penis if Viagra or the other medications do not work. These devices press against the body to form a closed space. Air is pumped out of the tube, and blood rushes into the penis to replace it. A rubber band is placed at the base of the penis to keep the blood inside. The band also blocks the flow of semen, however. It is kept on for up to 30 minutes.

Implanted devices

A semi-rigid rod can be implanted in the penis to produce a permanent erection. If a patient does not like having a permanent erection, an inflatable prosthesis, like a balloon, can be inserted. A pump that is placed in the scrotal sac has fluid that inflates the penis for intercourse.

Bottom line: A man with erectile dysfunction has plenty of choices so that he can have a satisfactory sex life despite this disability. But, of course, the best course of action is to avoid diabetes altogether so ED isn't an issue at all — at least until much later in life.

Part V
Avoiding or Reversing Prediabetes

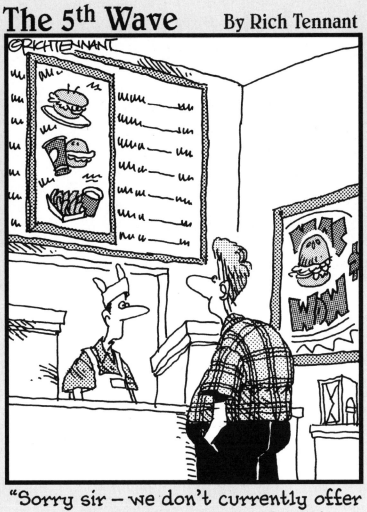

The 5th Wave   By Rich Tennant

"Sorry sir – we don't currently offer a 'Happy Hemoglobin Meal.'"

In this part . . .

Prediabetes does not have to turn into diabetes. This part shows you how to prevent that progression.

From shopping for food in a new way to cooking for health and enjoyment, I show you how to deal with your intake of calories. I also clearly demonstrate how to maximize movement so you can increase your output of calories.

If lifestyle changes alone don't stop prediabetes in its tracks, you have other alternatives: namely medications and surgery for weight loss. I tell you everything you need to know about these options.

I sum up all this advice with a chapter to get you moving in the right direction: a three-month program of diet, exercise, and behavior modification. Follow it carefully, and you will be well on your way to normal metabolism.

Chapter 15

Shopping for Food in a New Way

In This Chapter

▶ Studying your supermarket's layout

▶ Making more frequent trips to the store

▶ Getting to know each section of the store

▶ Becoming a label-reading expert

▶ Getting what you need for your pantry and fridge

The old way of shopping is not working. It has left you weighing more, feeling unhappy with the way you look, and staring at prediabetes: a prelude to diabetes if you don't do something significant. Poor food choices are one of the things that got you to this place. Good food choices will help to get you back where you belong: in a state of excellent health. Chances are, the place you choose most of your foods is the supermarket, so we're going to visit it in this chapter.

You may think of the supermarket as the place where you get the food that your body requires. The people who run the supermarket think of it as a place to maximize profits from the food it sells. So those people have done numerous studies, focus groups, and other learning experiences to pinpoint how to get you to spend more. One result has been the enormous consumption of unneeded calories and the development of obesity in so many people, leading to prediabetes and diabetes.

In this chapter, you find out how the supermarket is set up, how you can overcome its temptations, and how to use your supermarket for your good health. You discover everything a food label can tell you. You learn which ingredients to buy and which to pass by. Finally, I show you how to stock your pantry and refrigerator and have the tools you need to cook great food. By the end, you will be a truly informed shopper. You will be much wiser than baseball great Yogi Berra, who was once asked whether he wanted his pizza cut into four or eight pieces. "Better make it four," he said. "I don't think I can eat eight pieces."

Looking at the Grocery Store's Layout

All grocery stores are laid out the same way. The standard layout is not created for your convenience but to maximize sales. Basically, all the fresh, perishable items — the fresh fruits and vegetables; the fresh breads; and the meat, fish and poultry — are on the perimeter of the store. To get to the milk, for example, you either have to pass by all the fresh items and then go back again that way (which is the longest way around the store), or you have to go through the aisles, past all the enticing, expensive, canned and prepared foods that are filled with chemicals and preservatives. These aisle foods are also the high-calorie choices. You go by the candies, cookies, sugared cereals, and all the other no-nos.

To avoid buying the wrong foods, you must stick to the edges of the store, no matter how much longer your route to the milk is.

This layout is one of numerous techniques that grocery stores use to entice you to buy what you don't need but perhaps want. Here are some other tricks they use, and the ways you can circumvent them:

- ✔ Grocery stores are usually cold because you tend to buy more when you are cold. Go to the store dressed in layers so you aren't cold.

- ✔ All stores love credit cards, which you think of as expandable cash. Buy with cash if you can't avoid buying impulsive items.

- ✔ Grocery stores have the smell of fresh baked goods wafting throughout. You buy more when you smell good food. You must either resist the smells or wear some strong perfume or cologne that blocks them out.

- ✔ Grocery stores depend on you being hungry when you shop, because you buy much more under that circumstance. People tend to shop at just the wrong time, when they come home from work and are famished. Shop on a full stomach.

- ✔ Grocery stores fill the checkout area with high-calorie impulse foods. This is the place where you stand the longest, so you can't help but notice the candies and other items. To minimize this problem, shop when the store is least crowded so you zip right past them. That would be early morning or later at night after the commuting crowd has gone home.

- ✔ Grocery stores also give you easy access to convenience items. Don't buy them because they're usually too salty and too fatty. They are also fairly expensive, and you would do better making them yourself.

You can save up to 40 percent if you regularly make a shopping list and stick to it.

✔ Grocery stores run sales, which may seem like great deals. Remember that sale items are not always the best food for you, nor are they the cheapest way to buy food. So-called *loss leaders* are foods priced often below their cost to the market in order to entice you in, because supermarket gurus know you won't stop with that one purchase. Other sale items are usually discounted about 10 percent below their usual cost. *Phantom* sale items really offer little or no discount but are marked with a "sale" sign as though they did. Just keep in mind that saving money does not prolong your life.

Shop at the same market as often as possible so you become familiar with its marketing techniques.

✔ Grocery stores give away free samples. Don't be tempted by them because they're usually high in calories.

✔ Grocery store layouts try to direct you through the aisles, which feature canned and other processed foods. Buy foods in the following order: fresh, frozen, canned. Fresh are the best, but frozen are not far behind because food producers don't have to add preservatives to frozen foods. (Canned foods usually contain lots of salt.) If you can't get something fresh, you can usually buy it frozen. But fresh usually means in season, which means the greatest availability and the lowest prices.

✔ Grocery stores plant the worst food choices at "kid level." Don't bring your kids to the store if you can help it. If you must, make sure they aren't hungry, and don't allow them to take things off the shelves.

✔ Grocery stores love the colors red and yellow because they grab your attention. Avoid items packaged in red and yellow, or at least pay close attention to what exactly you're getting.

Your shopping basket contents should look like the types and amounts of foods that are recommended in the U.S. Department of Agriculture's Government Food Pyramid (see Chapter 16).

Shopping More Often

One of the best techniques for eating well is to eat fresh. That means going to the market regularly to get the freshest foods that are in season. When you eat fresh foods that are in season, you accomplish a number of things:

✔ You minimize the energy that is used to transport the food. (Some foods in your supermarket travel thousands of miles to reach you.)

✔ You get food that is just off the vine or the tree or out of the ground, when it contains the maximum amount of nutrients.

✔ You get more local food so you have a chance of knowing the farmer who grew it. You may even be able to know a farmer's philosophy of using compost or fertilizer or poison sprays for bugs.

✔ You get to know the people at the market who are a source of good advice and knowledge of what is available and when.

I could make numerous suggestions for ways to shop more often, but here are just a few:

✔ Shop at the best stores you can afford for the freshest produce, but buy only what you can use in the next few days so it doesn't spoil.

✔ Buy less food in general so you have to return to the store more often.

✔ Shop at farmers' markets, where the food is totally fresh, often picked that morning, and free of preservatives.

✔ Because you are not buying a lot each time and won't have much to carry, try to walk all or part of the way to the store to get some exercise.

When you shop more often, you also create a community of people that you meet at the market. These people not only become your friends but share recipes and tell you where they have found good food and good bargains.

Visiting the Sections of the Market

Each section of your supermarket presents a different challenge as you go through trying to stay with good nutrition. You need to use different shopping strategies in each department.

The bakery

The bakery is the home of the carbohydrate. Here you find all kinds of rich pastries, muffins, cookies, and other treats that are hard to resist. The large display cases full of delicious-looking cakes and pies beckon you like the Sirens of Greek mythology, who lured unwary sailors to their death.

Baked goods usually contain too much fat and too much carbohydrate. Some are made sugar-free for people with diabetes, but the other ingredients, especially the fats, more than make up for the lack of sugar. Others are made fat-free because people mistakenly believe that eating fat makes us fat. In truth, the total calories are what matter — not where they come from (see Chapter 6).

Compared to 1970, we are eating almost 50 percent more grains these days. But 90 percent of the grains we eat are refined grains (the bad kind), not whole grains (the good kind). One reason we're eating more grains these days is that the size of baked goods has grown enormously in the last 40 years. What was a whole bagel in the 1960s is now half a bagel. While you could get a muffin with 100 kilocalories in the 1960s, today you buy a muffin at least twice that size (with at least twice the number of calories, of course). Today, a blueberry muffin could have 510 kilocalories and 19 grams of fat. If you must buy muffins, bagels, and other baked goods, make two to three meals from them.

You don't have to give up baked goods completely, but stick to small portions. Save half a muffin for the next day, or share it with a friend. And choose baked goods with lots of fiber and fruits.

The produce department

Here is where you find fresh fruits and vegetables. Once upon a time, your fruit choices were limited to apples, oranges, bananas, and a few summer fruits. Now you can find all kinds of exotic fruits from exotic lands. Don't be afraid to try something new! These fruits can serve as dessert in place of bakery goods. Some of the new melons, for example, are very sweet and have a great texture.

Try many different vegetables as well. The different colors mean they contain different kinds (and amounts) of nutrients that you need. And vegetables, for the most part, are very low in calories. Even though we're eating more vegetables today than we did in 1970, we're still not eating sufficient quantities to satisfy the recommendations of the federal government.

If you love a particular type of seasonal fruit, you may be able to prolong its season by freezing the fruit: putting it into a freezer bag and using it as you need it. This process works especially well with berries, which can be frozen on a cookie sheet.

Dried fruits and fruit juices are better choices than many other snacks, but they aren't the same as the fresh stuff. Dried fruits are sources of very concentrated carbohydrates, and fruit juices are missing the important fiber. Stick to whole fruits and vegetables as often as possible.

The dairy case

Since 1970, we are eating 20 percent less dairy. The good news is that we're consuming less whole-fat milk and more low-fat milk. But our overall consumption of dairy products has fallen, which is unfortunate because dairy is a major source of calcium.

At the same time, up to 75 percent of adults suffer to a greater or lesser extent from a condition called *lactose intolerance.* This condition results from someone having an absence or reduction of *lactase,* an enzyme that breaks down *lactose,* a sugar that is present in milk and other dairy products. African Americans, Asian Americans, and Native Americans are especially susceptible to lactose intolerance. Outside the United States, the people of Asia, Africa, South America, and Latin America suffer the most. They develop the following symptoms:

- ✔ Bloating
- ✔ Cramping
- ✔ Diarrhea
- ✔ Flatulence
- ✔ Nausea

They lose their production of lactase and can't tolerate dairy products as adults, so they generally do not eat them.

If you can tolerate dairy products, try going for the low-fat varieties. (However, in certain circumstances, you can suspend that rule. For example, if you get the opportunity to go to France, eating low-fat cheese is almost silly. You are better off having full-fat cheese but very little of it.)

High-fat dairy products contain plenty of saturated fat. As I mention in Chapter 10, saturated fat is dangerous to your health. Keep the portions small.

The deli counter

Processed meats are dangerous to your health! They cause cancer, particularly pancreatic cancer and colon cancer. Avoid them! The culprit is probably the sodium nitrate in the meats. Processed meats include:

- ✔ Almost all red meat in frozen prepared meals
- ✔ Bacon
- ✔ Beef jerky

- ✔ Bologna
- ✔ Canned soups with meat
- ✔ Frozen pizza with meat
- ✔ Ham
- ✔ Hot dogs
- ✔ Pepperoni
- ✔ Salami
- ✔ Sausage

Meats in the deli section are usually heavily salted and contain too much fat, even without the cancer-causing sodium nitrate.

Salads in the deli area are another matter. They can be delicious and low-calorie convenience meals. They are fresh and appealing to the eye and the taste. But choose salads made with oil, not cream.

The meat and fish counter

Ounce for ounce, you find some of the most expensive food in the market here. The funny thing is that you are often paying the most for what may be the least healthy for you. People who eat meat are, on average, heavier than those who don't and have more diabetes as well.

Here are some specific suggestions for shopping in this part of the store:

- ✔ Buy more poultry and fish than red meat.
- ✔ Get exactly what you want in terms of ounces. Otherwise, you end up eating too much.
- ✔ Make sure the fish is wild, not farmed.
- ✔ If you must eat red meat, choose low-fat cuts like top round, sirloin, and flank steak.
- ✔ Buy skinless poultry to avoid the fat.
- ✔ Eat fish twice a week for the positive effect it has on your blood fats.
- ✔ Fish and meat may come breaded for your convenience, but don't buy it — there is too much butter fat in the breading.
- ✔ Fish that smells fishy is not fresh.

Lentils and other legumes are a good source of protein. You don't have to eat only meat, fish, or poultry to get protein.

Frozen foods and diet meals

This section of the supermarket offers both good choices and bad. One of the good choices is frozen vegetables. You can find your favorite vegetables in the frozen food section when the growing season is over. Food makers know how to lock in the flavor and don't need preservatives because the food is *flash frozen,* meaning rapidly frozen in very low temperatures. These veggies are easy to prepare with a few minutes in the microwave oven.

In contrast, the full meals you can buy frozen are usually bad choices. They're often extremely high in salt and fat, so be sure to check the food labels before putting them in your cart.

Diet frozen meals, however, tend to be lower in calories, salt, and fat. Not only that, but they taste pretty good. Healthy Choice, Lean Cuisine, and Weight Watchers are the main brands of diet meals. Healthy Choice tends to be lower in salt.

If you're choosy about what you buy and take the time to read the labels, frozen meals can be a decent choice when you have little time to prepare food. But if you like to prepare your foods and love the taste of fresh, make your own.

Canned foods

More than 1,500 food products are available in cans. Some canned foods, like tomatoes and other fruits, can be very convenient. But canned foods often contain a lot of oil, salt, and/or sugar. Again, you want to check the food labels to find out exactly what you're getting. You may be able to find low-sugar or low-salt varieties of your favorite canned foods, including soup.

Bottled drinks

While you're keeping a close watch on how many canned foods get in your cart, you may want to aim to keep the bottled drinks out altogether. The United States ranks first among countries in soft drink consumption. What a dubious honor! And what a waste of money! Soda has been called "liquid candy." Bottled soda and fruit juice drinks are high in sugar and low in nutrition. Here are some other facts about soft drinks:

✔ Many children begin to consume them as young as age 1 and 2.

✔ The biggest consumers are 12- to 29-year-old males, who drink more than two 12-ounce sodas daily.

✔ The soda industry has steadily increased the sizes of bottles and cans from 6.5 ounces in the 1950s to 20-ounce bottles today. The 6.5-ounce can had 5 teaspoons of sugar in it. The 20-ounce can or bottle has 17 teaspoons of sugar.

✔ The soda industry promotes excessive soda drinking by:

- Spending the largest advertising and marketing budgets for any type of product that is consumed. (I refuse to call soda "food.")

- Promoting concerts and sporting events.

- Providing vending machines in schools and giving a little of the money earned back to the schools.

- Creating tie-ins with popular movies like *Harry Potter* and *Star Wars*.

- Hiring star athletes to pitch their drinks.

- Coming up with new forms of soft drinks to target specific populations.

✔ Soda provides the average American with 7 teaspoons of sugar a day.

✔ Teenage boys and girls consume their recommended daily allowance for sugar in soda alone. Then they have fruit drinks, candy, cookies, cake, ice cream, and other sources of sugar. This problem alone is enough to explain the epidemic of obesity in this country.

✔ When someone consumes so much soda, little room is left for many other foods that contain important micronutrients. It's not surprising that soda drinkers consume far less fiber, vitamins, and calcium than they need.

✔ In addition to obesity, numerous health risks are associated with drinking excessive soda, even diet soda. They include:

- Osteoporosis from lack of calcium.

- Tooth decay and erosion.

- Heart disease because the high sugars promote the metabolic syndrome that I discuss in Chapter 9.

- Addiction to the caffeine in most soft drinks. Caffeine causes further loss of calcium in your urine. Plus, it affects your performance and mood.

My advice is that you treat the drink aisle of the grocery store as though it was selling poison. The only thing missing from bottles and cans of soft drinks is the skull and cross bones usually found on products that are meant to poison rats.

Instead of bottled soda or bottled water, try adding some lemon juice to plain tap water. Or put some water and strawberries in your blender and create a really delicious and low-cost beverage that quenches your thirst.

The snack aisle

What you eat between meals may make the difference between weight loss and weight gain, so you have to choose carefully. Be honest: Whatever you bring into your house is going to be eaten. If you know it's not good for you, don't tempt yourself. Here are suggestions for the best things to buy for snacks:

- ✔ Baked chips are much less fattening than fried chips.
- ✔ Celery and carrot sticks are an excellent, healthy choice free of calories.
- ✔ Flavored rice cakes can fill you up without the calories.
- ✔ Fruit and fig bars, like Fig Newmans, can satisfy your hunger while keeping the calories under control.
- ✔ Low-fat granola is much better than regular granola. Regular granola may provide twice as many calories.
- ✔ Plain popcorn, popped in an air-popping machine, has only 30 kilocalories per cup.
- ✔ Raisins and other dried fruits have concentrated calories, so keep the portions small.

Reading and Understanding Food Labels

In Chapter 4, I take a brief look at the food label. Now that we are in the grocery store, let's take a closer look. We're going to pick up a package of frozen peas and see what we can learn about the food in that package by reading the food label. Figure 15-1 shows what the label on a package of Trader Joe's Petite Peas looks like.

On the left side, you see the serving size, which, in this case, is 2/3 cup or 85 grams. You also find out the number of servings in the package: about five. The remaining information on the package all refers to the amount in *one serving,* so if you eat the whole package, you are getting five servings and you have to multiply all values by 5. Keep in mind that the serving size suggested on a food label may not be the same as the one in your food plan.

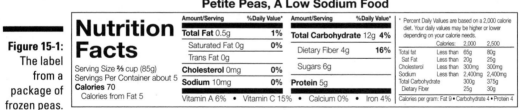

Figure 15-1:
The label
from a
package of
frozen peas.

Ingredients: Petite Peas

Here is the other specific information you find on a food label:

- ✔ **Total fat:** The total fat in one serving of peas amounts to 0.5 grams. But is that good or bad? To the right of the list of amounts per serving are the U.S. government recommended values for both a 2,000- and 2,500-calorie diet. A 2,000-calorie diet should contain less than 65 grams of fat, so 0.5 grams represents no more than 1 percent of that amount. That's very, very good.

- ✔ **Saturated fat and trans fat:** You want to keep your saturated fats low and your trans fats even lower (because they're the very worst kind of fats). In these peas, the percent of each is 0, which is terrific. Make your life easy: If you see trans fat listed on a food label, don't buy the product. And try to keep the saturated fat levels down as well.

- ✔ **Cholesterol:** Again, lower is better. This product contains no cholesterol, so the percent is 0. Always choose foods that are lower in cholesterol when you have a choice.

- ✔ **Sodium:** Sodium is a component of salt, and the sodium amount in this product is 10 mg. Because the daily recommendation is less than 2,400 mg, that value is essentially 0 percent. Unlike these peas, many prepared foods are high in sodium. Keep a close watch on the sodium content of the foods you eat, and choose the ones that are lower.

- ✔ **Total carbohydrate:** The total carbohydrate in one serving of peas is 12 grams, or 4 percent of the recommended value. That amount breaks down into 4 grams of fiber (16 percent of the daily recommended value) and 6 grams of sugar. The label doesn't explain where the other 2 grams of carbohydrate are located. The key here is to look for foods with more fiber and less sugar. Different diets recommend different percentages of carbohydrate, so there is no specific recommendation for daily carbohydrate consumption.

- ✔ **Protein:** The total protein in one serving of peas is 5 grams. There is no recommended value for protein on the label for the same reason there is no carbohydrate recommendation.

✔ **Vitamin and mineral content:** Toward the bottom of the label are the percentages of certain vitamins and minerals contained in one serving of this food. Vitamins A and C are reflected, along with calcium and iron. The reason these are chosen is that most Americans don't get enough of them in their diets. Choose foods with higher percentages whenever possible.

✔ **Percent daily value information:** To the right of the label, you find information called *percent daily value.* This information refers to how much of each component of a food you should eat based on a total 2,000-calorie diet. In general, if a food contains 5 percent or less of the daily value of a certain component (such as saturated fat or sodium, for example), that's low. If the food contains 20 percent or more of a component, that's high. If you get 20 percent of your fat from this food, for example, you can get the other 80 percent from all other foods you eat that day.

Just because the type of food is the same doesn't mean you'll get the same percent daily values in different packages with the same food in them. For example, one container of yogurt may have a very different amount of calcium from another. That's why reading food labels is always a good idea.

✔ **Ingredients:** The list of ingredients is very important so you can avoid foods with large numbers of ingredients and compare foods. This package contains only peas. If there were other ingredients, they would be listed in order by weight. Look for good ingredients like olive oil, canola oil, peanut oil, and whole grains. Avoid bad ingredients like high fructose corn syrup and chemicals with names you can't pronounce.

One serving of these peas provides about 70 kilocalories with just a few grams of sugar and protein. If you pick up some other brand of peas, you can compare the values on the label and choose the one with less calories, fat, and sodium.

Stocking the Essentials in Your Pantry and Fridge

You should keep a number of basic products in your pantry or refrigerator so that you can whip up a delicious meal at any time and know it will fit into your nutritional program. You can turn this list into a shopping list and just fill in what you need to buy so you get everything you need and nothing you don't need.

For the freezer:

- ✔ Chicken breasts
- ✔ Egg substitute
- ✔ Frozen fruit
- ✔ Frozen shrimp
- ✔ Frozen vegetables
- ✔ Fruit juice concentrate
- ✔ Loaf of whole grain bread

For the pantry:

- ✔ All natural peanut butter
- ✔ Canned fruit, unsweetened
- ✔ Canned tomatoes, no salt added
- ✔ Canned tuna or salmon in water
- ✔ Dried, unsugared fruit
- ✔ Evaporated skim milk
- ✔ Fat-free salad dressing
- ✔ Fresh garlic
- ✔ Fruit spreads
- ✔ Grains (brown rice, couscous, quinoa)
- ✔ Legumes (peas, beans, lentils)
- ✔ Mustard
- ✔ Nonfat dry milk
- ✔ Nonstick cooking sprays
- ✔ Oils (olive, canola, peanut)
- ✔ Onions
- ✔ Whole wheat pasta
- ✔ Pasta sauce
- ✔ Potatoes and sweet potatoes
- ✔ Red and white cooking wines
- ✔ Reduced-calorie ketchup

✔ Reduced-calorie mayonnaise

✔ Reduced-sodium broths

✔ Reduced-sodium soy sauce

✔ Sugar-free cocoa mix

✔ Tomato paste

✔ Vinegars

✔ Worcestershire sauce

For baking:

✔ Baking powder

✔ Baking soda

✔ Cocoa powder

✔ Cornstarch

✔ Cream of tartar

✔ Dry bread crumbs

✔ Extracts (vanilla, lemon, almond)

✔ Flour (all purpose, whole wheat)

✔ Rolled oats (not quick cooking)

✔ Semi-sweet chocolate

✔ Sugar-free gelatin

✔ Unflavored gelatin

Sweeteners:

✔ Artificial sweeteners

✔ Honey

✔ Light maple syrup

✔ Molasses

✔ Sugar

Seasonings:

✔ Dried herbs

✔ Fresh herbs and spices

✔ Pepper

✔ Salt

Using these ingredients and a few others that you buy only when you need them, you are ready for just about any recipe. If you like to cook a certain ethnic food, you may want to stock up on some basic ingredients specific to that type of food.

Obviously, you want to also buy perishables like fresh fruit and vegetables as they come into season, getting only as much as you need while they can stay fresh.

Using the Right Tools

Successful cooking requires the right pots, pans, knives, and so forth. In this section, I offer a list of the essentials for that purpose.

Get good quality equipment. You will use a knife over and over again, and if it's not good quality, you will eventually tire of it and get good quality anyway. You may as well start with excellent tools. The same is true for pots and pans. Nonstick pots and pans are such a pleasure to wash that you won't regret spending a bit more at the beginning.

Here are the key things you need:

- Chopping boards
- Food processor
- Knives of very good quality
- Measuring cups and spoons
- Microwave
- Mixer with dough hook
- Nonstick pots and pans
- Salad spinner
- Scales
- Steamer with double boiler
- Thermometers for roasts and turkey

Now you are set to make delicious foods like the recipes in the next chapter. Just watch your portions!

Chapter 16

Cooking and Eating for Health and Enjoyment

*W*hat you find in this chapter is the essence of what you need to know about avoiding diabetes and eliminating prediabetes. That's because what and how much you put into your mouth can get you into trouble. Keep in mind that not everyone with prediabetes and diabetes is eating the wrong things. Very often the problem is simply eating too much of the right things.

I make this point several times in this book (because it's crucial): When it comes to weight loss, the *total calories* you consume are what matter most, not so much where they come from. You may read all kinds of discussions about how protein is better because you burn it faster, how fat is better because it does not stimulate insulin, or how carbohydrate is better because it reflects the kind of diet our ancestors ate. But the fact is that whether people eat a diet high in protein, carbohydrate, or fat, if the calories are kept constant, they lose exactly the same amount of weight after a year.

Does that mean you should eat a high-fat diet for the next year? It does not. You would be missing all kinds of vitamins, minerals, and other essential foodstuffs. Instead, you want to eat a balanced diet with reduced calories so you lose the weight that is very likely the source of your problems but still consume all the essential foodstuffs that you need to keep your body healthy.

Chances are that you did not become heavy by eating massive amounts of food. Over time, by eating as little as 100 extra kilocalories a day (a little more than a slice of bread or a little less than a 12-ounce can of beer or a 6-ounce glass of wine), you may have gained 1 pound a month, which adds up as time goes by: 12 pounds a year, 24 pounds in two years.

The great news is that losing weight works exactly the same way as gaining it, just in reverse. By eating just 100 kilocalories less a day, you lose 1 pound a month, which also adds up over time. This chapter is all about how to get your weight loss started. Be sure to also check out Chapter 20, where I tell you the exact steps to take during the first three months of your journey toward better health.

Knowing What to Eat

A number of organizations have tried to make it easier for you to know what to eat. The major recommendations come from the U.S. government, the American Diabetes Association, and the American Heart Association. You would think that these entities would have exactly the same suggestions, but nothing in life is quite so simple. I point out the differences among their suggestions in this section. I follow up their recommendations with discussions of how to increase your fiber intake, make your meals more colorful, and much more.

Following the U.S. government food pyramid

The latest version of the U.S. government food pyramid is shown in Figure 16-1. The triangles in the pyramid represent the various kinds of foods you should be eating every day. From left to right, here's what the largest triangles represent: grains, vegetables, fruits, milk, and meat/beans. (For the moment, ignore the sliver triangle in the middle.) The size of each triangle indicates how much of your diet should be composed of that food. If you eat a 2,000-calorie daily diet, here's what the triangles mean:

- **Grains: Eat 6 ounces every day.** Eat at least 3 ounces of whole grain cereals, breads, crackers, rice, or pasta ever day. One ounce is about one slice of bread; ½ cup of breakfast cereal; or ½ cup of cooked rice, cereal, or pasta.

- **Vegetables: Eat 2½ cups every day.** Eat more dark green veggies like broccoli, spinach, and other leafy vegetables. Eat more orange vegetables like carrots and sweet potatoes. Eat more dry beans and peas, like pinto beans, kidney beans, and lentils.

- ✔ **Fruits: Eat 2 cups every day.** Eat a variety of fruits. Choose fresh, frozen, canned, or dried fruit. Go easy on fruit juices.

- ✔ **Milk: Get 3 cups every day.** Get low-fat or fat-free when you choose milk, yogurt, and other milk products. If you don't or can't consume milk, choose lactose-free products or other calcium sources such as fortified foods and beverages.

- ✔ **Meats and beans: Eat 5½ ounces every day.** Choose low-fat or lean meat or poultry. Bake it, broil it, or grill it. Vary your protein routine by choosing more fish, beans, peas, nuts, and seeds.

Now, back to that sliver triangle, which is fourth from the left in the pyramid diagram. The government recommends limiting our intake of sugars and salt (sodium), but it recognizes that we do need a small amount of fat in our diets. The sliver triangle represents oils, which can be a healthy source of fats if you choose the right kind. Olive, canola, and peanut oil are considered among the best kinds to choose. You want to avoid coconut and palm oils.

Most of the fat you eat should come from fish, nuts, and vegetable oils. Limit or eliminate altogether the solid fats you eat, like butter, margarine, shortening, and lard. Read nutrition labels to avoid saturated and trans fats.

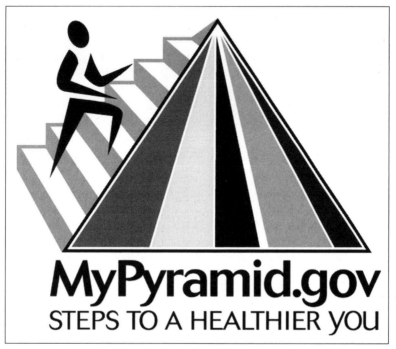

Figure 16-1:
The U.S. government food pyramid.

If you are wondering what the person is doing on the steps on the government pyramid, he (or she) is there to emphasize the importance of exercise in a healthy lifestyle. For my exercise recommendations, be sure to turn to Chapter 17.

The U.S. government has gone to an enormous amount of trouble to make the food pyramid useful. You can find lots of valuable resources at `www.my pyramid.gov/pyramid/index.html`:

- ✔ **Inside the Pyramid** allows you to click on the parts of the pyramid to get more information. For example, if you click on the second triangle from the left, a discussion of vegetables pops up, describing the five subgroups of vegetables based on their nutrient content: dark green vegetables, orange vegetables, dry beans and peas, starchy vegetables, and other vegetables.

- ✔ **Tips and Resources** offers tips to make the food pyramid easier to use. For example, "Get your calcium rich foods" moves you to the milk section while "Keep food safe to eat" tells you how to prepare cooked foods to the proper temperature and how to keep your work surfaces clean.

- ✔ **Got a Question?** lets you know that you can call someone at the My Pyramid Customer Support Line (888-779-7264; open from 8 a.m. to 3 p.m. Eastern time, Monday through Friday) or send an e-mail to `support@cnpp.usda.gov`.

- ✔ **MyPyramid Plan** allows you to customize the food groups based on your height, weight, gender, age, and amount of physical activity. It notes whether you are the proper weight for your height. If you are overweight, it permits you to choose a food plan for your current weight or to gradually move toward a healthier weight. Then it allows you to print out a PDF version of your results. Twelve different versions of the food pyramid are available depending on your height, weight, and level of activity.

- ✔ **Menu Planner** gets into the specifics of the foods you need to eat. You can fill in the details of the foods you plan to eat, and it will tell you whether or not you are following the correct plan.

- ✔ **Child Cost Calculator** allows you to estimate how much it will annually cost to raise a child.

- ✔ **MyPyramid Podcasts** links you to audio presentations on all aspects of the Food Pyramid, as well as physical activity. If you learn better by listening, be sure to check out this feature.

MyPyramid also addresses specific audiences with recommendations for their particular needs. These include:

- ✔ Preschoolers
- ✔ Kids
- ✔ Pregnant and breastfeeding women

I highly recommend this Web site for all the valuable information. If you aren't online already, this site is a good reason to get connected.

Checking out American Diabetes Association guidelines

The American Diabetes Association (ADA) recommends various ways to follow a healthy diet that avoids both prediabetes and diabetes. In addition to recommending the U.S. government food pyramid, ADA also promotes two methods called *creating your plate* and *carbohydrate counting.*

Creating your plate

Creating your plate is exactly what it sounds like. It involves setting up your meal plate to improve your nourishment and decrease your calories. These are the steps you take:

✔ Put a line down the middle of your plate with a marker. (I recommend not using your finest china.)

✔ On one side of the plate, put another line down the middle. You've now created two smaller sections and one larger section.

✔ Fill the largest section with non-starchy vegetables including beets, broccoli, bok choy, cabbage, carrots, cauliflower, cucumber, green beans, greens, lettuce, mushrooms, okra, onions, peppers, salsa, spinach, tomatoes, turnips, and vegetable juice.

✔ In one of the small sections, put starchy foods like

- Cooked beans and peas, such as pinto beans or black-eyed peas

- Cooked cereal like oatmeal, grits, hominy, or cream of wheat

- Whole grain breads such as whole wheat or rye

- Whole grain, high fiber cereal; low-fat crackers and snack chips; pretzels; or fat-free popcorn

- Potatoes, green peas, corn, lima beans, sweet potatoes, or winter squash,

- Rice, pasta, dal, or tortillas

✔ In the other small section, put meat or meat substitutes like

- Chicken or turkey without the skin

- Fish such as tuna, salmon, cod, or codfish

- Lean cuts of beef or pork

- Other seafood like shrimp, clams, oysters, mussels, or crab

- Tofu, eggs, or low-fat cheese

✔ Add an 8-ounce glass of non-fat or low-fat milk. If you don't drink milk, add 6 ounces of light yogurt or a small roll.

✔ Add a piece of fruit or ½ cup of fruit salad.

The result will be something very similar to the recommendations for the food pyramid. Although fats don't have a place on the plate, they can be used for cooking. Occasionally, sweets can replace other starchy foods or fruit, but only in small portions. If you want a snack, save your milk or fruit for between meals.

Counting carbohydrates

The other suggestion of the ADA is to count carbohydrates so that you eat about 45 to 60 grams of carbohydrate at a meal. Because carbohydrates raise blood glucose, limiting yourself to this much carbohydrate decreases the amount of insulin secreted in your body.

Following are a number of foods that contain 15 grams of carbohydrate. You can choose three or four of them to make up your plate:

✔ 4 ounces of fresh fruit

✔ ½ cup of canned fruit or frozen fruit

✔ One slice of bread (preferably whole grain)

✔ ½ cup of oatmeal or cream of wheat

✔ ⅓ cup of pasta or rice

✔ ½ cup of black beans or starchy vegetables

✔ 3 ounces of baked potato

✔ ⅔ cup of plain, fat-free yogurt

✔ 1 cup of soup

If you consume about half your daily calories this way, the other 50 percent should be 30 percent fat and 20 percent protein. You will eat about 50 grams of fat and 75 grams of protein to round out this diet.

Considering American Heart Association suggestions

The American Heart Association (AHA) is much more fat-conscious than the government or the ADA because excessive fat, especially *saturated fat* (found in animal protein) and *trans fats* (added by food manufacturers), can do more than cause weight gain: It causes increased cholesterol and *arteriosclerosis,* which is the blockage of critical arteries, especially to the heart. The AHA warns against the Bad Fats Brothers, Sat and Trans, and encourages the Better Fats Sisters, Mon and Poly. Its food recommendations include the following:

✔ Use up at least as many calories as you take in.

✔ Eat a variety of nutritious foods from all the food groups, especially vegetables and fruits.

✔ Choose whole grain, high fiber foods.

✔ Consume fish, especially oily fish, at least twice a week.

✔ Eat fewer nutrient-poor foods, such as beverages and foods with added sugars, foods with trans fats or saturated fats, foods with a lot of sodium, and foods high in cholesterol.

✔ Consume alcohol only in moderation.

✔ Avoid tobacco in any form, active or passive.

Increasing fiber

Fiber is the part of a carbohydrate that is not digestible, so it adds no calories. You find fiber in fruits, grains, and vegetables. Fiber comes in two forms:

✔ **Soluble fiber** can dissolve in water. It tends to lower blood glucose and fat levels, especially cholesterol.

✔ **Insoluble fiber** can't dissolve in water so it remains in the intestine, where it absorbs water and stimulates movement, preventing constipation and colon cancer. This type of fiber is called *bulk* or *roughage*.

You don't find fiber in refined foods or in animal sources of food. The daily recommendation for fiber is 20 to 30 grams, which is more than most people eat. You should try to increase your fiber uptake, but do so slowly to avoid triggering diarrhea. If you currently eat very little fiber and try to eat 30 grams tomorrow, the results could be explosive.

Table 16-1 shows the fiber content of various foods.

Table 16-1	Foods' Fiber Content	
Fruits	*Serving Size*	*Fiber (Grams)*
Apple with skin	1 medium	8.0
Banana	1 medium	3.1
Blueberries	1 cup	3.5
Figs	2 medium	3.7
Orange	1 medium	3.1
Pear with skin	1 medium	5.1
Raisins	1.5-ounce box	1.6
Raspberries	1 cup	8.0
Strawberries	1 cup	3.3
Grains, Cereals, and Pasta	*Serving Size*	*Fiber (Grams)*
Barley, cooked	1 cup	6.0
Bran flakes	¾ cup	5.1
Bread, rye	1 slice	1.9
Bread, whole wheat	1 slice	1.9
Brown rice, cooked	1 cup	3.5
Oat bran muffin	1 medium	4.0
Oatmeal, quick or cooked	1 cup	5.2
Popcorn	3 cups	3.6
Spaghetti, whole wheat, cooked	1 cup	6.3
Legumes, Nuts, and Seeds	*Serving Size*	*Fiber (Grams)*
Almonds	1 ounce (22 nuts)	3.3
Baked beans, cooked	1 cup	10.4
Black beans, cooked	1 cup	15.0
Lentils, cooked	1 cup	15.6
Lima beans, cooked	1 cup	13.2
Pecans	1 ounce (19 halves)	2.7
Pistachio nuts	1 ounce (49 nuts)	2.9
Split peas, cooked	1 cup	16.3
Sunflower seeds	¼ cup	3.6

Vegetables	Serving Size	Fiber (Grams)
Artichoke	1 medium	10.3
Broccoli, boiled	1 cup	5.1
Brussels sprouts, cooked	1 cup	4.1
Carrot, raw	1 medium	1.7
Peas, cooked	1 cup	8.8
Potato with skin, baked	1 medium	4.0
Tomato paste	¼ cup	2.7
Sweet corn, cooked	1 cup	4.6
Turnip greens, boiled	1 cup	5.0

Creating a colorful plate

You need a variety of fruits and vegetables in order to eat all the micronutrients you need in your diet. Eating fruits and vegetables with different colors is a good approach. Here are some of the different colored fruits and vegetables and what nutrients they provide:

- ✔ **Blue and purple** foods include blackberries, blueberries, eggplant, grapes, plums, prunes, and purple varieties of fruits and vegetables like cabbage, figs, and raisins. The color comes from anthocyanins. Within these purple treats are vitamin C, fiber, ellagic acid, and quercetin.

- ✔ **Green** foods include artichokes, asparagus, avocado, broccoli, Brussels sprouts, celery, cucumbers, green apples, honeydew, leeks, lettuce, limes, onions, peas, spinach, sugar snap peas, and zucchini. The green derives from the natural plant pigment chlorophyll and provides fiber, calcium, vitamin C, and beta-carotene, which lower blood pressure, improve cholesterol, improve your eyes, and protect against cancer.

- ✔ **Red** foods include apples, beets, cherries, cranberries, grapes, onions, papaya, pears, peppers, pink grapefruit, radishes, raspberries, strawberries, tomatoes, and watermelon. The red color comes from three antioxidants — lycopene, ellagic acid, and quercetin — as well as hesperidin, another substance that protects against cancer.

- ✔ **White** foods include bananas, cauliflower, corn, garlic, ginger, jicama, mushrooms, nectarines, onions, peaches, potatoes, and turnips. The white color is from anthoxanthins. These contain beta-glucans, SDG, and lignans that boost your immune system, reduce your cancer risk, and balance your hormones. They also provide potassium.

> ✔ **Yellow and orange** foods include apricots, butternut squash, cantaloupe, carrots, grapefruit, lemon, nectarines, oranges, peaches, pineapples, sweet corn, sweet potato, tangerines, and yellow varieties of many other fruits and vegetables. The yellow comes from beta-carotene and vitamin C, which protect your eyes, improve your bones, and fight cancer.

Isn't Mother Nature generous? The least you can do is acknowledge her generosity by partaking of her bounty. Here are some suggestions for doing so:

✔ Add raisins to your morning oatmeal.

✔ Add raspberry jam to your morning toast.

✔ Drink a ½ cup of orange juice at breakfast.

✔ Have lettuce, tomato, and onion on your lunch sandwich.

✔ Enjoy a cup of vegetable soup for lunch.

✔ Have several mini carrots on the side of your lunch.

✔ Eat a snack of apple slices.

✔ Enjoy steamed broccoli and cauliflower for dinner.

✔ Have a spinach salad.

✔ Feast on angel food cake with blueberries for dessert.

✔ Eat a banana snack.

You will add lots of micronutrients that you need and few calories that you don't need.

Sticking with food you can recognize

One of the simplest rules you can follow that will prevent you from eating things that may not be good for you is to stick to foods you can recognize as food. Anything that has more than three or four ingredients is not simple, basic food; it is a concoction created by chemists, not Mother Nature.

Let's take an example. I walked into a 7-Eleven and purchased a box of Nissin Cup Noodles with Shrimp. These are the ingredients listed on the label:

Enriched flour (Wheat flour, niacin, reduced iron, thiamine mononitrate, riboflavin, folic acid), Vegetable oil (Contains one or more of the following: Canola oil, cottonseed oil, palm oil, rice oil), Preserved by Tocopherols and/or TBHQ and/or Ascorbyl Palmitate, Salt, Dehydrated Vegetables (Carrot, Green Pea), Freeze-dried Shrimp, Soy Sauce Powder (Wheat, Soybeans, Maltodextrin, Salt), Monosodium Glutamate, Hydrolyzed Soy, Corn and Wheat Protein, Spices, Caramel Color,

Potassium Carbonate, Sodium Carbonate, Sodium Tripolyphosphate, Pork Powder, Garlic Powder, Natural Flavors, Chicken Powder, Sodium Alginate, Disodium Succinate, Dissodium Guanylate, Disodium Inosinate, Shrimp Powder, Autolyzed Yeast Extract, Cod Liver Oil.

Now I don't know about yours, but my grandmother never heard of 95 percent of these ingredients, much less ever used them. What do they provide for this "food"? They provide artificial color, artificial flavor, and artificial duration of shelf life. Just like the mummies in Egypt that are intact after 2,000 years, these "foods" may be edible in 2,000 years. Food was not meant to last 2,000 years or it would come with preservatives built in! While the preservatives help this concoction to last a long time on the shelf, I am not so sure they were meant to enter our bodies.

Let's try another example. Here are the ingredients on a can of Campbell's SpaghettiOs with Meatballs purchased at a Walgreen's pharmacy. (Perhaps the fact that I bought this product at a pharmacy should have made me realize I was buying chemicals.)

Water, Tomato Puree (Water, Tomato Paste), Meatballs (Beef, Pork, Water, Bread Crumbs, Enriched Flour [Wheat Flour, Niacin, Ferrous Sulfate, Thiamine Mononitrate, Riboflavin, Folic Acid], Dextrose, Salt, Yeast, Soybean Oil, Soy Protein Concentrate, Salt, Dehydrated Onion, Dehydrated Garlic, Beef Flavor [Beef Stock, Flavoring, Salt, Spice Extract]), Enriched Macaroni Product with added Calcium and Vitamin D (Wheat Flour, Calcium Phosphate, Niacin, Ferrous Sulfate, Thiamine Mononitrate, Riboflavin Folic Acid), Contains less than 2% of Sugar, Carrot Juice Concentrate, Salt, Enzyme Modified Cheddar Cheese (Cheddar Cheese, Cultured Milk, Salt, Enzymes, Calcium Chloride), Water, Disodium Phosphate, Enzymes, Potassium Chloride, Vegetable Oil, Enzyme Modified Butter (Milk), Yeast Extract, Flavoring, Ascorbic Acid, Citric Acid, Nonfat Dry Milk, Malic Acid, Succinic Acid.

I remember visiting my grandmother as a boy, and my mother asked my grandmother to go easy on the Malic Acid and the Disodium Phosphate in the spaghetti and meatballs. No, just kidding. This is not food! It's another chemical feast. We have to stop eating these things and go back to basics.

If you count five or more ingredients on a food label, put it back on the shelf.

Taking the glycemic index into account

All carbohydrates are not alike in the degree to which they raise the blood glucose. This fact was recognized some years ago, and a measurement called the *glycemic index* was created to quantify it. The glycemic index (GI) uses white bread as the indicator food and assigns it a value of 100. Another carbohydrate of equal calories is compared to white bread in its ability to raise the blood glucose and is assigned a value in comparison to white bread. A food that raises glucose half as much as white bread has a GI of 50, and a food that raises glucose 1½ times as much has a GI of 150.

A study reported in the November 2007 *Archives of Internal Medicine* showed that in a group of Chinese women who tended to eat a lot of high glycemic index rice, there was a significant increase in the risk of developing type 2 diabetes. Another study in the same issue showed that increasing the level of low glycemic cereal in the diet reduced the risk of type 2 diabetes in a group of African American women, a group that is getting type 2 diabetes in epidemic numbers.

The benefits of low glycemic index foods are numerous. Many of them are exactly what you need to prevent prediabetes from turning into diabetes. Here are some of the things low glycemic foods can do:

- Help people lose and control their weight
- Increase insulin sensitivity
- Reduce heart disease risk
- Reduce cholesterol
- Reduce hunger
- Prolong physical endurance

The point is to select carbohydrates with low GI levels to try to keep your glucose response as low as possible. A glycemic index of 70 or more is high; 56 to 69 is medium; and 55 or less is low.

The following complications have caused the GI to be underutilized:

- The GI of a carbohydrate may be different when it is eaten alone or as part of a mixed meal.
- The GI of a food may differ if it's processed and prepared differently.
- Some low GI foods, like chocolate, contain a lot of fat.
- Diabetes educators have been reluctant to teach the GI concept because they believe it is hard to understand and will create confusion.

However, good clinical studies have shown that knowledge of the GI of food sources can be very valuable. Evaluation of the diets of people who develop diabetes compared with those who don't shows that, all other things being equal, the people with the highest GI diet most often develop diabetes. After diabetes is present, those who eat the lowest GI carbohydrates have the lowest levels of blood glucose. Patients in these studies have not had great

difficulty changing to a low GI diet. The other thing that happens whei
GI food is incorporated into a diet is that the levels of triglycerides an_ _ _
(bad) cholesterol fall.

I believe that switching to low GI carbohydrates can be very beneficial for controlling your glucose and avoiding diabetes. You can easily make some simple
substitutions in your diet, as shown in Table 16-2.

Table 16-2	Simple Low GI Substitutions
High GI Food	*Low GI Food*
Whole meal or white bread	Whole grain bread
Processed breakfast cereal	Unrefined cereals like oats or processed low GI cereals
Plain cookies and crackers	Cookies made with dried fruits or whole grains like oats
Cakes and muffins	Cakes and muffins made with fruit, oats, and whole grains
Tropical fruits like bananas	Temperate climate fruits like apples and plums
Potatoes	Pasta or legumes
White rice	Basmati or other low GI rice

Because bread and breakfast cereals are major daily sources of carbohydrates,
these simple changes can make a major difference in lowering your glycemic
index. Foods that are excellent sources of carbohydrate but have a low GI
include legumes such as peas or beans, pasta, grains like barley, parboiled
rice and bulgar, and whole grain breads.

Even though a food has a low GI, it may not be appropriate because it is too
high in fat. You need to evaluate each food's fat content before assuming that
all low GI foods are good for you.

Likewise, even though a food has a high GI, it may still be acceptable in your
diet if it contains very little total carbohydrate. For example, cantaloupe has
a GI of about 70, but the amount of total carbohydrate is so low that it does
not raise your blood glucose significantly when you eat a normal portion.
This concept is called the *glycemic load* (GL), a number that takes both glycemic index and total carbohydrates into account.

If you want to go into this subject in deeper detail, you can find a listing of
many foods by category of food, portion size, and level of GI and GL on the
Web at www.glycemicindex.com.

Reducing Your Fat Intake

Especially if you have a problem with cholesterol, you can take many steps to reduce the fat in your diet without ending up with something as bad or worse. (See the sidebar "Beware the low-fat promise.") Here are some of the best tricks for keeping the fat out of your mouth:

✔ Read labels and don't buy the food if the fat content is over 30 percent or the saturated fat content is over 10 percent.

✔ Never buy food with *trans fats,* also known as *partially hydrogenated oils.* That includes margarines.

✔ Substitute lean beef, fish, poultry, fruits, vegetables, beans, and other legumes for higher fat meats and cheeses.

✔ Trim all visible fat from beef or poultry and remove the skin.

✔ Bake, broil, or roast; never deep-fry. Use lemon juice or low-fat broth for moisture and flavor.

✔ Use spices rather than fat for flavor.

✔ Pan-fry or use a wok with small amounts of oil.

✔ Use as little butter as possible.

✔ Don't eat fatty gravies. If you must have them, put them on the side of your plate and use them sparingly.

✔ Use fat-free or 1 percent milk and low-fat dairy products.

✔ Use two egg whites and one yolk in place of two whole eggs.

✔ Avoid vegetable oils that are harmful, like palm and coconut oil.

✔ Substitute yogurt for sour cream.

✔ Avoid high-fat nuts like coconuts and macadamia nuts.

✔ Use low-fat lunch meats rather than salami or bologna. Avoid bacon, hot dogs, and other sausages.

✔ Make sure your salad dressing is made with unsaturated oils.

✔ Skim off the fat from soup prepared the day before.

✔ Eat home-baked cookies prepared with less fat.

✔ Make air-popped popcorn without butter.

✔ Eat fresh fruit in place of high-fat desserts.

Beware the low-fat promise

It seems obvious that because fat has twice as many calories per gram as protein or carbohydrate, simply removing fat from your diet will result in significant weight loss and improvement in your insulin sensitivity. Watch out! That may not be the case. Remember, it's the total calories that count, not the number of fat calories.

Food manufacturers add a lot of sugar to make up for the absence of fat. While fat has a certain filling quality that causes you to stop eating because it is slowly absorbed, sugar is rapidly absorbed, and you tend to eat a lot more. So just because a food is low in fat does not mean that it is nutritious. In order to get you to buy diet foods, the manufacturers try to make them seem like the high-fat foods you are trying to avoid. The result is the addition of a lot of artificial colors and flavors that are not food.

Remember: You want to make a change in your food preferences — not just substitute chemical foods for real foods. Substitute foods that work for you for foods that don't. (See the discussion of the glycemic index in this chapter for examples.)

Hydrating Your Body

I talk frequently in this book about the evils of soft drinks, which are often called *liquid candy*. You want to avoid soft drinks at all costs, but you also want to make sure you substitute plenty of healthy liquids. All cells and organs in your body require water. The best liquid around, the one that makes up 70 percent of your body, is water.

Water has many important functions in your body. For example, water

- ✔ Acts as the carrier for blood cells, oxygen, food, and breakdown products of metabolism
- ✔ Acts as a lubricant around your joints
- ✔ Regulates your body temperature
- ✔ Prevents and alleviates constipation
- ✔ Helps to absorb shocks to the brain
- ✔ Enhances fat loss
- ✔ Reduces hunger
- ✔ Makes you look younger by hydrating your skin

You can buy water that is more expensive than gasoline, or you can turn on the cold-water faucet in your house and drink from there. In the United States, tap water is as good as water from any other source. Some people prefer to filter their water. If you're one of them, you can attach an inexpensive filtering device to your spout, and the water is collected below in a storage box. An *activated carbon filter,* for example, will treat taste and odor problems.

Water is essential for life. You can live a long time without food, depending on how much energy you have stored in your body, but you can't live more than a few days without water. Your body is constantly losing water that must be replaced. The daily losses include:

- 28 to 40 ounces in breath and perspiration
- 20 to 55 ounces from urination
- 2 to 7 ounces in your stool

The recommendation you often hear is to drink eight 8-ounce glasses of water daily. But what if you lose the maximum amount of water each day just through breathing, perspiring, urinating, and passing stool? You could lose as much as 102 ounces a day. Drinking 64 ounces of water may not be enough. Underhydration could explain a lot of the muscle symptoms people get, especially cramps.

A different way to determine your daily need for water is to take your weight and divide by two. If you weigh 150 pounds, you need about 75 ounces of water a day.

If you are feeling hungry, drink water. The hunger pangs may go away or at least decrease. If you like a little taste in your water, try making citrus water:

- 1 gallon of water
- 1 large lemon, sliced
- 1 large orange, sliced

Combine and chill for two hours. Strain out the fruit and enjoy.

Another way to get plenty of water is to eat food that contains a lot of it. Some of the best sources of water in food include:

- Broccoli
- Cabbage
- Cauliflower
- Grapefruit
- Honeydew melon
- Lettuce
- Radishes

> ✔ Spinach
>
> ✔ Watermelon

Some people have had great success losing weight with the *BDA* diet. They drink 8 ounces of water *before, during,* and *after* each meal. Doing so results in significant weight loss and reduction in hunger. And it's a lot less expensive than weight loss surgery!

Changing Your Pace and Your Portions

The way we eat has a lot to do with how much we eat. Many behavioral scientists believe that we would have much better control over our calorie intake if we changed our approach to food. Of course, portion control is essential if we are to reduce our food intake. This section contains suggestions for using these techniques to reduce your weight and prevent prediabetes from becoming diabetes.

Modifying your eating behavior

Having worked with overweight and obese patients for years, I know that diet and exercise alone do not keep weight off; some fundamental changes in eating behavior are required. And believe me, you want to make it as easy as possible to keep weight off for the long haul.

Eating even a little bit of the things you know are not good for you usually doesn't work because you can't stop at one. For example, you know that the muffins you buy in a bakery are much larger than one serving. You tell yourself that you will buy a muffin, cut it in half, and leave the other half for tomorrow. Doing so may work once or twice, but it won't work consistently. You will eat that whole muffin just as you will overeat at a buffet. It is far better to avoid exposure to temptation than to depend on willpower to get you through.

Here are some changes you can make in your eating behavior that avoid the necessity for willpower:

> ✔ **Eat according to a schedule to avoid unplanned eating.** Eat three meals a day and two or three snacks daily, preferably at the same time each day. The snacks should be low in calories, such as carrot sticks or celery.
>
> ✔ **Find a single place to eat all your food.** This is a "designated eating place," where all you do is eat. It should not be your desk, where you do many other things.

- ✔ **Slow down your eating to make the meal last.** Put down your fork or spoon between each bite, and don't pick it up until you have swallowed the food. Chew each bite for a long time.

- ✔ **Use smaller plates and shallow bowls to reduce the size of your portions.** You will be amazed at how quickly you will be satisfied with less food.

- ✔ **Do nothing but eat when you are eating.** No TV, Web surfing, talking on the phone, or reading allowed.

- ✔ **Keep all food in the kitchen.** Don't leave plates of food on counters. Keep leftovers in opaque containers.

- ✔ **Put high-calorie foods away.** Remove serving dishes and bread from the table.

- ✔ **Don't dispense food to others.** Also, don't serve meals family style.

- ✔ **Do not clean your plate.** If you can learn to leave food on your plate, you may learn to stop eating when you are full.

- ✔ **Set realistic goals for weight loss.** A goal of a few pounds in a week or a month is much more doable than talking about 60 pounds.

- ✔ **Keep a diet journal.** List the foods you're eating, the amount and type of exercise you've done, and what mood you're in.

- ✔ **Eat fresh fruit for dessert.**

- ✔ **Avoid fast food as much as possible.**

- ✔ **Take special care in restaurants.** When eating out, be careful of salad dressing (ask for it on the side), alcohol (have a maximum of one drink), and bread (try to keep it off your table altogether).

- ✔ **Add water to your diet.** As I explain earlier in the chapter, drinking lots of water could be one of the best of your new eating behaviors.

- ✔ **Carry around a 10-pound weight.** Doing so can help you appreciate the importance of losing that much weight.

- ✔ **Reward your success with non-food items.** Think about movies, CDs, or books, for example. You can give yourself a money prize (perhaps a dollar) every time you do something for your health, like passing up loose candy in the market or Cinnabon at the airport. When the money adds up, purchase something you have really wanted.

- ✔ **Never eat from emotion.** Many people overeat because they have learned that food makes them "feel better." If that describes you, remember that the good feeling is very temporary, and ultimately, the extra food will hurt your health. Try to break the connection between food and feelings.

- ✔ **Get seven to eight hours of sleep nightly.** Sufficient sleep reduces appetite.

- ✔ **Be a disciplined shopper.** At the market, buy from a list, carry only enough money for the food on that list, and avoid aisles containing loose foods other than fruits and vegetables.

Incorporate one of these techniques into your life at a time. After you feel you have mastered it and have added it to your eating style, take up another technique.

Remember that you are human and not a robot. You will screw up, but your mistakes need not be fatal. Just get back to the habits that you know will work.

As you go about this difficult task of losing weight and keeping it off, remember to seek the help of those around you. A loving partner provides great help through the roughest days.

Reducing portions

As I note earlier in the chapter, a good way to start reducing your portions is to use smaller plates and bowls to eat from. Here are some other techniques for reducing portions:

- ✔ Make a rule to eat no more than half your usual portion whether at home or in a restaurant. Doing so will cut your calories in half. When you eat out, always take food home.

- ✔ Stick to the right size portion. For example, a serving of meat is the size of a deck of cards, and a serving of pasta is the size of a tennis ball.

- ✔ Never eat seconds!

- ✔ Never eat straight from the bag, box, or carton. There's no telling how much you will eat under those circumstances.

- ✔ Put away leftovers before you eat so that they are not tempting you.

- ✔ Always check the food labels to discover the serving size. You may be surprised that a can that looks like one serving is actually intended for two. If you eat the whole thing, you may be consuming way too many calories.

Keeping a Food Record

Keeping a food record has proved to be one of the most reliable and valuable ways to understand why you are not losing weight and what you have to do to start losing. I have had numerous patients come to me with the same refrain: "I can't lose weight!" It takes just a few days of keeping a food record to understand why this is so.

Don't wait until the end of the day to write down what you've eaten. Many studies have shown that our memory is not reliable (or perhaps we don't *want* to recall every bite we've taken). Write down the food at the time you eat it.

Keep track not just of the type of food but also of the portion size. Also write down how much exercise you do each day, and make notes about your mood or feelings.

You may want to use a free weight loss and diet journal online, such as FitDay (www.fitday.com). After you have signed up, you keep a log of the foods you are eating. For example, if you choose meat, the FitDay site gives you the choice of the type of meat: pork, beef, and so on. When you choose beef, the site asks for the cut of beef and how it was cooked. After you provide all the details, you click on "Add to Food Log." You keep track of your exercise and mood in a similar fashion. You can also record your body measurements if you desire.

At FitDay, you can create numerous reports about your food and activity to help you get a sense of your progress. For example, you can create

- ✔ A pie chart that shows how many calories you've eaten that day, which breaks down calories from fats, protein, and carbohydrate.
- ✔ A report on your average daily intake for all nutrients, including all the vitamins and minerals. (You can even get your average daily nutrition displayed as a nutrition facts label.)
- ✔ Your nutrition as a percentage of the recommended daily allowance of various vitamins and minerals.
- ✔ A graph of your average daily calories over time.
- ✔ A pie chart that shows how much saturated, polyunsaturated, and monounsaturated fat you're eating.
- ✔ A pie chart that shows your average daily calories burned.

This list is just a sample. You may be amazed at the number of tools available to you for free, whether online or as an application on your BlackBerry or iPhone. If you are the kind of person who likes to fill in the blanks, this kind of tool could be the way for you to go.

Always share your food record information with your doctor. The two of you can discover together why you may be having trouble losing weight.

Trying Some Simple Meal and Snack Recipes

So let's do a little cooking. I want to provide you with some simple and delicious meal and snack recipes that were given to me by some of the best chefs in America. We tried them, changed them to make them more nutritious if necessary, and ran them by the chefs to make sure we hadn't made unacceptable changes. Try them for yourself, and be sure to check out my *Diabetes Cookbook For Dummies,* 2nd Edition (Wiley) for many more suggestions.

Breakfast

People who diet successfully always eat breakfast. In fact, they don't skip any meal, but eat lightly at each meal. Try these recipes if you don't generally eat much breakfast. They will change your habits.

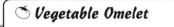 Vegetable Omelet

Enjoy this omelet for breakfast or any other time of day when you want a satisfying little meal. It's easy to prepare. Add fresh, seasonal vegetables, and perhaps some fresh herbs, for maximum nutrition.

Preparation time: *10 minutes*

Cooking time: *10 minutes*

Yield: *4 servings*

Nonstick cooking spray	*2 broccoli florets*
½ medium zucchini	*4 whole eggs*
4 mushrooms	*8 egg whites*
½ bell pepper	*1 medium plum tomato, seeded and chopped*

1 *To prepare vegetables:* Cut zucchini and pepper into thin strips. Cut mushrooms into quarters and finely chop onion. Chop broccoli florets.

2 Coat a large skillet (preferably nonstick) with cooking spray and place over medium heat. Sauté vegetables, stirring often, until tender.

3 In a bowl, mix together eggs and egg whites and season with pepper. Pour egg mixture over vegetables in skillet. Add tomatoes to skillet. Cover pan and cook over low heat until eggs are cooked and puffy, 5 to 7 minutes. Serve immediately.

Per serving: 134 calories, 15 grams protein, 6.7 grams carbohydrate, 5.5 grams fat, 1.6 grams saturated fat, 212 milligrams cholesterol, 2 grams fiber, 183 milligrams sodium.

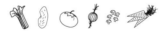

☞ Breakfast Pizza

As any cook knows, eggs can be served in so many ways: incorporated into salads, added to sauces and meatloaf, and in this recipe, used as the filling for an inventive sandwich that was inspired by the pleasures of pizza. A small amount of shredded cheese is made to stretch, supplying plenty of flavor without all the calories of your favorite fast food!

Preparation time: *15 minutes*

Cooking time: *20 minutes*

Yield: *4 servings*

1 loaf French or Italian bread	*4 whole eggs*
Nonstick cooking spray	*8 egg whites*
1 tablespoon unsalted butter	*4 medium red potatoes, boiled, diced small*
½ small onion, finely chopped	*½ cup shredded, reduced-fat cheddar cheese*
½ teaspoon garlic powder	
1⅛ teaspoon black pepper	

1 Preheat oven to 350 degrees Fahrenheit.

2 Cut bread in half, lengthwise. Scoop out half of soft center. Place bread, crust cut side up, on a baking sheet covered with cooking spray, and spread bread with butter.

3 Coat a large well-seasoned or nonstick skillet with the cooking spray and place over medium heat. Sauté onions stirring often, until tender, about 5 minutes. Spray the pan again with oil if necessary and add potatoes, garlic powder, and pepper. Sauté for 5 minutes.

4 In a bowl, whisk together eggs and egg whites. Add to onion–potato mixture. Cook over medium heat, stirring to scramble until eggs are cooked.

5 Spoon egg mixture into bread. Sprinkle cheese on top. Bake 8 to 10 minutes until cheese melts. Cut each half of the bread in half again, crosswise. Serve immediately.

Per serving: 447 calories, 25 grams protein, 58 grams carbohydrate, 13 grams fat, 5.5 grams saturated fat, 225 milligrams cholesterol, 4 grams fiber, 632 milligrams sodium.

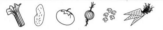

Lunch

Salad used to be a side dish, but creative chefs have turned it into a main course. Here are a couple of salads: one that will serve as a nice side dish with a bowl of soup, and the other that can be a full lunch.

⌒ Simple Green Salad with Citrus and Herbs

The dressing in this salad makes use of regular lemons and naturally sweet Meyer lemons. If Meyer lemons aren't available, substitute with ruby red grapefruit, which adds rosy color. Enjoy this salad with some cheese and crackers for a light but balanced meal.

Preparation time: *15 minutes*

Cooking time: *None*

Yield: *4 servings*

Tahini dressing:

¼ cup freshly squeezed Meyer lemon juice or ruby red grapefruit juice

2 tablespoons freshly squeezed lemon juice

2 teaspoons finely sliced fresh chives

1 tablespoon finely sliced fresh chervil

1 teaspoon finely sliced flat parsley leaves

¼ cup lemon oil

¼ Meyer lemon segments or ruby red grapefruit segments, divided use

¼ teaspoon salt and freshly ground pepper to taste

The salad:

1 head Bibb or Boston lettuce

4 cups loosely packed baby greens or baby lettuce

1 In a medium mixing bowl, make the dressing by combining the Meyer lemon juice, regular lemon juice, chives, chervil, parsley leaves, lemon oil, and half the Meyer lemon segments.

2 Separate the leaves of the Bibb or Boston lettuce from the head. Gently wash them, keeping them whole; dry gently and set aside. Place the baby greens or baby lettuce in a medium mixing bowl.

3 Stir the dressing well and drizzle enough over the baby greens or baby lettuce to lightly moisten. Gently toss the greens until well covered.

4 Brush each Bibb or Boston lettuce leaf with some of the dressing. Arrange the four largest leaves in the center of four chilled salad plates. Mound some of the baby greens atop the Boston leaves. Place the next largest leaves atop the baby greens. Repeat until you have three layers of Boston lettuce leaves with the final layer covered with baby greens.

5 Place the remaining Meyer lemon segments around the salad.

Per serving: 153 calories, 2 grams protein, 11 grams carbohydrate, 14 grams fat, 1 gram saturated fat, 0 milligrams cholesterol, 4 grams fiber, 154 milligrams sodium.

☺ Jicama and Belgian Endive Salad with Tequila-Orange Vinaigrette

In this salad, orange sections add color, while jicama provides a satisfying crunch. Jicama is a bulbous root vegetable, native to Mexico, and has a sweet, nutty flavor.

If you omit the tablespoon of dressing over the endive leaves, you cut the fat in half. If you need to avoid alcohol, you can alter this recipe by substituting lime juice for the tequila.

Preparation time: *35 minutes*

Cooking time: *None*

Yield: *6 servings*

The vinaigrette:

¼ cup fresh orange juice

2 tablespoons tequila

1 tablespoon white wine vinegar

½ small shallot, peeled and chopped

¼ cup corn oil

¼ cup extra-virgin olive oil

½ teaspoon salt and freshly ground white pepper to taste

The salad:

2 medium jicamas, peeled and julienned

Chives, snipped for garnish

2 heads Belgian endive, rinsed, dried, and leaves separated

3 oranges peeled with a knife and sections removed

1 *To make the vinaigrette:* Place the orange juice, tequila, vinegar, and shallot in a blender and blend at high speed for 10 seconds.

2 Slowly add the oils through the opening in the lid while still blending. Blend for 10 or 15 seconds.

3 Add salt and white pepper.

4 *To assemble the salad:* On each plate, arrange the endive leaves, tip pointing out. Scatter the orange sections over the endive.

5 Toss the jicama with 6 tablespoons of the vinaigrette and mound in the middle of each plate. Ladle 1 tablespoon of the vinaigrette over the endive on each plate and sprinkle with the chives.

Per serving with 2 tablespoons dressing: 268 calories 2 grams protein, 29 grams carbohydrate, 16 grams fat, 2 grams saturated fat, 0 milligrams cholesterol, 13 grams fiber, 125 milligrams sodium.

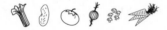

Dinner

Dinner is when the protein is served. In order to eat some healthful, nourishing protein, why don't we try some fish? Here are a couple recipes that are delicious and not too complicated.

Barbecued Tuna

This tuna steak recipe may be enjoyed with a homemade salsa prepared with roasted tomatoes. While fresh tuna can be pricey, you can substitute salmon to fit into your weekly budget.

Preparation time: *15 minutes*

Cooking time: *5 minutes*

Yield: *4 servings*

½ teaspoon ground cumin

½ teaspoon ground coriander

½ teaspoon ground white pepper

½ teaspoon ground black pepper

½ teaspoon fennel seed

1 tablespoon sugar

1 tablespoon chili powder

1 tablespoon paprika, sweet or hot

¼ teaspoon dry mustard

4 6-ounce tuna steaks

Olive oil as needed

1 *To prepare barbeque spice mixture:* In a small bowl, combine cumin, coriander, white pepper, black pepper, fennel seed, sugar, chili powder, paprika, and dry mustard, and mix thoroughly.

2 Brush tuna steaks lightly with olive oil and evenly dust on one side with barbecue spice mixture.

3 Brush nonstick sauté pan lightly with olive oil and heat over medium to high heat. Add tuna steaks, spice side down, and sear them for 1 to 2 minutes on the first side until lightly browned and spices form a crust. Turn steaks over, lower heat, and cook another 3 to 4 minutes for medium rare. Serve immediately.

Per serving: 230 calories, 40 grams protein, 3 grams carbohydrate, 5 grams fat, 1 gram saturated fat, 76 milligrams cholesterol, 0 grams fiber, 210 milligrams sodium.

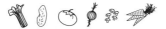

Lemon Sole with Brussels Sprouts

Here's a chance to get some good fish and some good vegetables in one dish. There is room for some potato or rice, as well as a roll or piece of bread, to round out this low-calorie meal.

Preparation time: *30 minutes*

Cooking time: *20 minutes*

Yield: *4 servings*

2 6-ounce filets of sole or flounder	*4 tablespoons grapeseed oil*
2¼ teaspoon of salt and pepper to taste	*1 teaspoon butter*
2 tablespoons salt	*1 tablespoon chopped shallots*
1 cup Brussels sprouts, trimmed and quartered	*¼ teaspoon thyme leaves*
	½ teaspoon chopped chives
1 tablespoon Dijon mustard	*Juice of 1 lemon*
2 tablespoons Champagne vinegar or white wine vinegar	

1 Preheat oven to 400 degrees Fahrenheit.

2 Season sole fillets with salt and pepper and place in baking dish lined with lightly greased foil.

3 Bring 6 quarts water and 2 tablespoons salt to a boil. Add Brussels sprouts and cook 3 to 4 minutes, until tender. Drain and refresh in the ice water. Drain again.

4 Mix Dijon mustard and vinegar in small bowl. Add salt and pepper if desired. Whisk in oil and set aside.

5 Heat butter in medium sauté pan, then add shallots and thyme. Cook for one minute, add Brussels sprouts and cook, tossing or stirring, for 2 to 3 minutes. Stir in the chives and remove from the heat. Cover loosely to keep warm.

6 Bake sole fillets for 6 to 8 minutes in the oven. Check for doneness by probing a filet at the thickest part with the tip of a paring knife — the flesh should be opaque inside and pull apart.

7 Place the Brussels sprouts in the center of each of four plates. Place the fish on top of the sprouts and squeeze several drops of lemon juice on the fish. Serve immediately.

8 Spoon the Dijon-vinegar-oil mixture around the plate.

Per serving: 237 calories, 17 grams protein, 4 grams carbohydrate, 16 grams fat, 43 milligrams cholesterol, 1 gram fiber, 255 milligrams sodium.

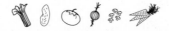

Is a vegetarian diet the way to go?

More and more evidence is accumulating that a vegetarian diet may be one of the healthiest diets that you can follow. Studies of Seventh-Day Adventists, some of whom follow a strict vegetarian diet and others of whom eat meat, showed that the meat eaters tended to be heavier and have more diabetes, high blood pressure, and high cholesterol on average. The American Dietetic Association published a position paper in the July 2009 edition of the *Journal of the American Dietetic Association* that says:

> *It is the position of the American Dietetic Association that appropriately planned vegetarian diets, including total vegetarian or vegan diets, are healthful, nutritionally adequate, and may provide health benefits in the prevention and treatment of certain diseases. Well-planned vegetarian diets are appropriate for individuals during all stages of the lifecycle, including pregnancy, lactation, infancy, childhood, and adolescents, and for athletes. A vegetarian diet is defined as one that does not include meat (including fowl) or seafood, or products containing those foods. . . . The results of an evidence-based review showed that a vegetarian diet is associated with a lower risk of death from ischemic heart disease. Vegetarians also appear to have lower low-density lipoprotein cholesterol levels, lower blood pressure, and lower rates of hypertension and type II diabetes than non-vegetarians. Furthermore, vegetarians tend to have a lower body mass index and lower overall cancer rates*

What do you think? Is vegetarianism the way to go for you? Keep in mind that even vegetarianism is not all gravy (pun intended). It is possible for a vegetarian to be obese if she eats enough fatty foods and carbohydrates.

Snacks

Here are a couple of simple snacks to provide those in-between calories without a lot of hassle:

- Two crackers and a small wedge of cheese
- A slice of apple and five almonds
- A small scoop of tuna salad and six grapes
- A slice of turkey on a rye crisp with a bit of mustard
- A smear of peanut butter on a couple slices of banana

Chapter 17

Maximizing Movement

In This Chapter

▶ Following government guidelines for exercise

▶ Starting out with walking

▶ Adding other exercises to the mix

▶ Investing in a pedometer

▶ Looking for incentives

▶ Doing resistance training exercises

Exercise is not an option; it's a necessity. If you've been living under the mistaken impression that you were given more than 640 muscles for no particular reason, allow me to clarify: Those muscles were put in your body for many reasons, the major one being to move your body through space. The more you move your body — and the more vigorously you move it — the healthier you will be. The old saying is absolutely true: If you exercise, you add life to your years and years to your life.

And exercise may improve more than just your physical health. One of my patients came in six months ago complaining of depression, so I gave her the name of a psychological therapist. When my patient returned recently, I asked how she was doing. She said that she was doing much better mentally. I asked if the therapist had helped her. She said that instead of seeing the therapist, she had greatly increased the amount of swimming that she was doing. She believed that the increased exercise had significantly improved her mental state.

If you have prediabetes, you have every reason to develop an exercise program. Such a program can not only head off the development of diabetes but can actually help you return to a healthy state, free of prediabetes.

In this chapter, you find out all you need to know to create your own exercise program. You learn the government's exercise recommendations, as well as my recommendations. You'll come to realize that you have many choices of types of exercise, several of which you may enjoy. You just have to choose what to do — and then do it!

Aerobic versus anaerobic exercise

When people talk about exercise, they often use the terms *aerobic* and *anaerobic* to distinguish two types. Briefly, here is what each term means:

✔ *Aerobic exercise* can be sustained for more than a few minutes, uses major groups of muscles, and gets your heart to pump faster during the exercise, thus training the heart. I give you many examples of aerobic exercise throughout this chapter.

✔ *Anaerobic exercise* is brief (sometimes a few seconds) and intense and usually cannot be sustained. Lifting large weights is an example of an anaerobic exercise. A 100-yard dash is another example.

Both types of exercise are important for long-term health.

What is the likelihood that you will make a change and adhere to it? The fact that you were motivated to buy this book is a good indication that you'll succeed. However, the odds of adhering to healthy lifestyle changes have fallen over the last ten years. A study that was published in *The American Journal of Medicine* in June 2009 compared how many U.S. adults adhered to healthy lifestyle habits in 1988 and 2006. The study looked at eating five daily servings of fruits and vegetables, exercising regularly (more than 12 times a month), maintaining normal weight, drinking alcohol in moderation, and not smoking. Adherence to all five healthy habits dropped from 15 percent of people in the National Health and Nutrition Examination Survey in 1988 to 8 percent of people in 2006. Please help to turn those statistics around!

Knowing U.S. Government Recommendations — and Mine

In 2008, the Centers for Disease Control and Prevention (CDC) of the U.S. government published its *2008 Physical Activity Guidelines for Americans.* The guidelines include recommendations for adults, children, older adults, and healthy pregnant or postpartum women. I outline the recommendations for each group in this section, and then I put in my own two cents.

For adults

Adults need at least:

✔ Two hours and 30 minutes (150 minutes) of moderate-intensity aerobic activity (such as brisk walking) every week and

✔ Muscle-strengthening activities on two or more days a week that work all major muscle groups (legs, hips, back, abdomen, chest, shoulders, and arms)

Or

✔ One hour and 15 minutes (75 minutes) of vigorous-intensity aerobic activity (such as jogging or running) every week and

✔ Muscle-strengthening activities on two or more days a week that work all major muscle groups

Or

✔ An equivalent mix of moderate- and vigorous-intensity aerobic activity and

✔ Muscle-strengthening activities on two or more days a week that work all major muscle groups

For **even greater health benefits,** adults should increase their activity to five hours of moderate-intensity aerobic activity or two hours and 30 minutes of vigorous-intensity aerobic activity per week plus the recommended muscle-strengthening activities.

For children

Children and adolescents should do 60 minutes or more of physical activity each day. The physical activity should include all of the following:

✔ Aerobic activity, which should make up most of your child's 60 or more minutes of physical activity each day. This can include either moderate-intensity activity such as brisk walking or vigorous-intensity activity such as running. Ideally, you want your child doing vigorous-intensity activity at least three days per week.

✔ Muscle-strengthening activities, such as gymnastics or push-ups, at least three days per week as part of the 60 or more minutes.

✔ Bone-strengthening activities, such as jumping rope or running, at least three days per week as part of the 60 or more minutes.

The CDC has created BAM! Body and Mind, a Web site designed for kids 9 to 13 years old to help them make healthy lifestyle choices. Go to www.bam. gov/sub_physicalactivity/index.html to check it out.

Determining how hard you're exercising

One way to determine how hard you're exercising is to measure your pulse and compare it to your target heart rate. To identify your target heart rate, the recommendation used to be that you would subtract your age from 220 and multiply the result by 60 percent and 75 percent. The resulting numbers provided the recommend range of heart rates during aerobic exercise.

More recent studies show that people can actually sustain aerobic exercise at higher heart rates, so your heart rate is no longer the only (or best) way to determine if your exercise is sufficient. The younger you are, the faster your exercise heart rate may be. If you are a world-class athlete training for your ninth marathon, your exercise heart rate may be higher.

So how do you determine if you're exercising at the right level of intensity? You can use the Perceived Exertion Scale. Using this scale, you give your exercise a descriptive value ranging from *very, very light* to *very, very hard* with *very light, fairly light, somewhat hard,* and *very hard* in between. You want to exercise to a level of *somewhat hard,* and you will be at your target heart rate in most cases. As you get into shape, the amount of exertion that corresponds to *somewhat hard* will increase.

Here is a description of these various levels of exercise:

- ✔ **Extremely light exercise** is very easy to do and requires little or no exertion.

- ✔ **Very light exercise** is like walking slowly for several minutes.

- ✔ **Light exercise** is like walking faster but at a pace you can continue without effort. This is equivalent to moderate-intensity exercise.

- ✔ **Somewhat hard exercise** is getting a little difficult but still feels okay to continue. This is equivalent to vigorous-intensity exercise.

- ✔ **Very hard exercise** is difficult to continue. You have to push yourself, and you're very tired. At this level, you have trouble talking. The very hard level of exercise is most beneficial.

- ✔ **Extremely hard exercise** is the most difficult exercise you've ever done.

Remember: Do not continue exercising if you have tightness in your chest, chest pain, severe shortness of breath, or dizziness.

For older adults

Older adults should follow the adult guidelines if possible. If doing so is not possible due to limiting chronic conditions, older adults should be as physically active as their abilities allow. The goal is to avoid inactivity. Older adults should do exercises that maintain or improve balance if they are at risk of falling.

If you're working with an older adult who can sit but cannot stand or walk, here are some ideas of how to proceed:

- ✔ Gradually remove arm support by starting with both hands holding on, then one hand holding on, then none.

✔ Then make the seating surface less stable by using a therapy ball.

✔ Gradually add upper extremity exercises like reaching and throwing.

✔ Then add manual resistance where the person has to pull.

If the older adult can stand but not walk, the progression to exercise is similar:

✔ Start by decreasing the amount of support from a walker to a cane to no device if possible.

✔ Move from standing on two legs to one.

✔ Make the surface less stable by making it irregular.

✔ Add steps.

✔ Introduce movement.

✔ Increase the speed of movement.

For the older adult who can walk, the progression is similar:

✔ Gradually reduce the use of any support.

✔ Make the walking surface more irregular.

✔ Increase the speed of movement and add changes in direction.

You don't need to get all your daily exercise at one time. For example, if you want to exercise 30 minutes on any given day, you may divide that goal into three ten-minute periods.

For healthy pregnant and postpartum women

Exercise is very important during a pregnancy and after delivery. It keeps your heart and lungs healthy during and after the pregnancy and improves your mood during the postpartum period. After delivery, exercise helps with weight loss. These are the CDC guidelines for this group of women:

✔ Healthy women should get at least 150 minutes per week of moderate-intensity activity, such as brisk walking, during and after their pregnancy.

✔ Healthy women who already do vigorous-intensity activity (such as running) or large amounts of activity can continue doing so during and after their pregnancy.

If you begin physical activity during your pregnancy, start slowly and increase your amount gradually over time. Avoid activities that involve lying on your back or that put you at risk of falling or abdominal injury, such as horseback riding, soccer, or basketball.

My recommendations

Although the CDC suggests that you can do either moderate-intensity activity or vigorous-intensity activity, I believe the evidence is overwhelming that vigorous-intensity activity is much more beneficial. An article in the *American Journal of Cardiology* in November 2006 looked at studies that compared the heart-protective benefits of moderate-intensity activity versus vigorous-intensity activity when the total energy expenditure was the same. The conclusion was that if the energy expenditure is held constant (for example, you walk twice as fast for half the time), exercise performed at vigorous intensity conveys greater protection for the heart than exercise at moderate intensity.

In other words, if the output of energy is the same, vigorous-intensity exercise provides the most benefits for your blood pressure, blood fats, and loss of body fat.

Starting a Walking Program

You have to walk before you can run. Walking is the easiest, least expensive, and most popular exercise there is. It requires only some good shoes and a safe place to walk. If you don't know how to walk for exercise, simply put one foot in front of the other and continue to do so for a minimum of 30 minutes. (An hour is even better.) If possible, walk with a partner; your time spent exercising will be much more pleasant.

If you've read many chapters in this book already, you probably think, "Dr. Rubin is never satisfied." And you're right. After you have proved that you can walk safely and comfortably for a minimum of 30 minutes, I want you to start to push yourself. Following are three walking programs for different starting fitness levels.

If you have been inactive or are overweight, follow this program:

Week	Walks Per Week	Distance (Miles)	Minutes Walking
1	3	.75	15
2	3	1.0	20
3	3	1.0	20
4	4	1.25	25
5	4	1.25	25
6	4	1.5	25
7	5	1.5	25
8	5	1.75	30
9	5	1.75	30
10	5	2.00	30

If you are physically fit and already exercising, use this program:

Week	Walks Per Week	Distance (Miles)	Minutes Walking
1	4	1.25	25
2	4	1.25	25
3	4	1.50	30
4	5	1.75	32
5	5	2.0	36
6	5	2.25	38
7	5	2.50	42
8	5	2.75	44
9	5	3.0	48
10	5	3.25	50

If you are already in excellent physical condition, consider this program:

Week	Walks Per Week	Distance (Miles)	Minutes Walking
1	4	2.0	35
2	4	2.0	35
3	4	2.25	39
4	5	2.50	43
5	5	2.75	47
6	5	3.0	51
7	5	3.25	51
8	5	3.50	53
9	5	3.75	56
10	5	4.0	60

Choosing Other Activities

While walking offers tremendous benefits, you may get bored if that's all you do for exercise. The best choice of an exercise for *you* is one that you enjoy and will continue to do. The choices are almost limitless, but keep in mind that more vigorous exercise is preferable.

After you start exercising, you definitely want to continue. Consider this motivation: If you've been exercising regularly and you stop, it takes only about two to three weeks to lose some of the fitness that your exercise has provided. And it can take up to *six weeks* to get back to that level of fitness. Try to keep exercising no matter the circumstances!

Figuring out your preferences

If you can't figure out what kind of exercise appeals to you, here are some suggestions that should help:

- ✔ Do you like to exercise alone or with company? Pick a competitive or team sport if you prefer company.

✔ Do you like to compete against others or just yourself? Running and walking are sports you can do alone.

✔ Do you prefer vigorous or less vigorous activity? Although more vigorous exercise is more healthful, any exercise is preferable to none.

✔ Do you live where you can do activities outside year-round, or do you need to exercise inside for much of the year? Find a sports club if weather prevents year-round outside activity.

✔ Do you mind investing in special equipment? If you don't want to invest much money, focus on walking and running so your only expense is a pair of good shoes.

✔ What benefits are you looking for in your exercise? Are you aiming mostly for cardiovascular conditioning, strength, endurance, flexibility, or body fat control? You should probably aim for all these benefits, but you may have to combine activities to get them all in.

Table 17-1 shows the benefits from various kinds of activity. You may need a combination of several of them to get all the benefits that exercise can provide.

Table 17-1	Match Your Activity to the Results You Want
If You Want to . . .	**Then Consider . . .**
Build up cardiovascular condition	Vigorous basketball, racquetball, squash, cross-country skiing, handball
Strengthen your body	Weightlifting (using low weights and high repetition), gymnastics, mountain climbing, cross-country skiing
Build up muscular endurance	Gymnastics, rowing, cross-country skiing, vigorous basketball
Increase flexibility	Gymnastics, judo, karate, soccer, surfing
Control body fat	Handball, racquetball, squash, cross-country skiing, vigorous basketball, singles tennis

You can tell from Table 17-1 that living in the mountains where you have plenty of snow is helpful because cross-country skiing is in almost every list. On the other hand, so is vigorous basketball, so you don't have to give up exercise if you live in a warm climate like Florida.

Cross-training, where you do several different activities throughout the week, is a good idea. Cross-training reduces the boredom that may accompany doing one thing day after day. It also permits you to exercise regardless of the weather because you can do some things indoors and some outdoors.

No matter what activity you choose, it's important to warm up and cool down for five minutes before and after you exercise. One way of doing so is stretching. Another way is simply to do your exercise at a lower level of intensity for five minutes before and after your workout.

Focusing on calories

If weight loss is one of your goals, you need to focus on calories: eating fewer and using more. Table 17-2 lists a variety of activities, including some that don't exactly fit into the category of *exercise* but offer some interesting comparisons. Next to each activity, I include the amount of kilocalories that you burn in 20 minutes.

Table 17-2	Kilocalories Burned from 20 Minutes of Various Activities	
Activity	*Kilocalories Burned If You Weigh 125 Pounds*	*Kilocalories Burned If You Weigh 175 Pounds*
Standing	24	32
Walking, 4 mph	104	144
Running, 7 mph	236	328
Gardening	60	84
Writing	30	42
Typing	38	54
Carpentry	64	88
House painting	58	80
Baseball	78	108
Dancing	70	96
Football	138	192
Golfing	66	96
Swimming	80	112
Skiing, downhill	160	224
Skiing, cross-country	196	276
Tennis	112	160

Everything you do burns calories. Even sleeping and watching television use 20 kilocalories in 20 minutes if you weigh 125 pounds.

Staying Active while Traveling

After you begin an exercise program you should make every effort to stay active when you travel. Doing so has a number of advantages:

- ✔ You will be more alert in a different time zone if you exercise.

- ✔ You will acclimate to the new time zone faster.

- ✔ You will be able to try the different foods at the new location without feeling you are overeating.

- ✔ You won't lose your fitness benefits.

Here are some of the things you can do to maintain your exercise while traveling:

- ✔ Find accommodations that have a fitness facility.

- ✔ Make use of the local parks and trails by reading about them in travel books before you go.

- ✔ Make sure you take the right attire like sneakers, gym shorts, and socks.

- ✔ Use every opportunity to exercise: Walk up stairs, walk to your meetings, and walk while you wait at the airport, for example.

- ✔ Don't try to improve your fitness on a trip; just maintain it.

- ✔ Plan time for fitness into your daily agenda.

- ✔ Reduce your exercise intensity and duration, especially if you have to use equipment that you are not familiar with.

Using a Pedometer

A *pedometer* is a little device you wear on your belt that counts the steps you take. It's one of the least expensive and most useful devices you can buy to assist your exercise program.

Buying the right kind

Pedometers are getting fancier and fancier, and they're getting increasingly more expensive as a result. Pretty soon they'll have built-in cell phones and music players. You don't need that kind of pedometer. All you need is a simple pedometer that accurately counts the steps you take. It shouldn't cost much more than $20 or $25.

The accuracy is important. You can test a pedometer by taking 100 steps and reading the result on your pedometer. It should be accurate within 5 percent, meaning you lose only 5 steps or less for every 100 you take. It can be tremendously frustrating to use a device that counts steps incorrectly.

Here are some of the other features that pedometers currently offer:

- Calories burned
- Distance calculation
- Pulse rate reader
- Seven-day memory
- Speed estimator
- Stopwatch
- Time of day
- Timer

In my opinion, all these features just complicate the pedometer and probably make it last a shorter time.

The accuracy of pedometers does fall off with time. In one study of three different pedometers, one was no longer accurate after six months, a second was no longer accurate after a year, and a third maintained its accuracy for more than four years.

The one that retained its accuracy the longest was the Yamax SW-200 Digiwalker Pedometer. It seems to be the gold standard of pedometers and simply gives you the number of steps. If you can, buy this one. Another option that is just as accurate (but at three times the price) is the New-Lifestyles NL-2000. After those two, accuracy falls precipitously.

If you want to know the distance you have walked, take ten normal steps and measure the distance you have gone. Divide that distance by ten to get your *stride length,* the distance you travel with each stride or step. Then multiply your stride length by the number of steps you take on any day to get the distance you have walked.

If you want to know the calories you have burned, your best bet is to find out the calories burned in a minute for a given exercise and multiply that number by the number of minutes you exercise. You don't want to rely on a pedometer for that measurement because it does not take into account your weight. In either case, you'll get an approximation, but the first method is more accurate.

Aiming for 10K a day

A surefire way to know that you have done enough exercise each day is to walk until you have a reading of 10,000 steps on your pedometer. For most people, that number represents a distance of 4 miles. That may seem like a huge, unattainable goal for you, but you may be surprised at how quickly you can reach it.

Begin by doing your usual amount of exercise each day. At the end of each day, record the steps you've taken and reset the number on your pedometer to zero. After seven days, add up the steps and divide by seven to get your daily count. You will probably find that you are doing between 3,000 and 5,000 steps a day.

Next, you want to build up your daily number. Here are some tips to help:

- ✔ Get a good pair of walking shoes or sneakers and replace them when they begin to wear out.

- ✔ Leave your car parked. If you can make a trip in an hour or less by foot, save your gas money and add substantially to your daily step count.

- ✔ Try to add a few hundred steps a week. Begin by identifying a baseline day in your first week when you did the most steps, and make every day like that one. Each week, add a few hundred more.

- ✔ Find an exercise buddy to walk with you. It's much more fun.

- ✔ Keep a record of the number of steps involved in various walks you take, so you can get the steps you are missing on any given day.

- ✔ Use stairs instead of the elevator, whether you're going up or down.

- ✔ Take a walk at lunchtime daily.

- ✔ Stop if you feel pain, and check with your doctor before continuing.

If you don't have a pedometer, you can go in the other direction to determine if you have done 10,000 steps. Use the following conversions:

- ✔ 1 mile = 2,100 average steps
- ✔ 1 block = 100 average steps
- ✔ 10 minutes walking = 1,200 steps on average
- ✔ Biking or swimming = 150 steps per minute
- ✔ Weightlifting = 100 steps per minute
- ✔ Rollerskating = 200 steps per minute

Keep in mind that the more vigorous the exercise, the greater you'll benefit —
even when doing 10K a day. Try to do your steps vigorously!

Like all great ideas, the plan of 10K a day has gotten some bad press. It is not
based on any particular research. However, to get 10K a day, you would generally have to exercise more than 30 minutes and up to 60 minutes, which is
the recommendation of the CDC. If you want to lose weight but are not doing
so with 10K, do 12K or 14K. Keep in mind that 10K should not be the maximum you aim for, but rather the minimum. For more information on the value
of more steps, see *The Step Diet* by James O. Hill, Ph.D. (Workman Publishing
Company).

Getting Awarded and Trekking the Country

You may be the kind of person who likes tangible rewards for doing your
exercise, or you may want to feel you are actually going somewhere as you
walk the same 4 or 5 miles each day. If so, keep reading.

Taking the President's Challenge

If you like tangible rewards for what you do (besides the rewards of lower
blood glucose, lower cholesterol, lower blood pressure, and possibly lower
weight), join the President's Challenge at www.presidentschallenge.org.
The Web site provides a place to record your activity, and it offers all kinds
of information on activities for every age. You choose what you like to do,
and every time you do it you record your progress.

The beginner's program is called the Active Lifestyle Program. Here's what
you do:

1. **Choose an activity.** Any activity that uses large muscle groups counts.
   Adults need to do at least 30 minutes of activity daily. Children under 18
   need to do at least 60 minutes of activity daily. The Web site lists almost
   100 different kinds of activity that are acceptable.

2. **Get active.** You have up to eight weeks to complete the program. The
   activity goals are in minutes or steps. The goal is 30 minutes daily for
   adults and 60 minutes daily for kids under 18 at least five days a week,
   for six out of eight weeks.

3. **Track your activity.** You can use the activity log on the Web site, or you can download a form so you track your progress on paper.

4. **Order your award.** When you have reached your goal, the activity log will remind you that you have earned an award that can be ordered online or by mail.

The Presidential Champions program is for people who are already active. You get activity points for everything you do, and you get more points for more vigorous activity. After you earn enough points you get the Presidential Champions bronze award. With still more points you get the silver award and eventually the gold award.

If you still want to do more and are active more than an hour a day, you would select the Advanced Performance Presidential Champions program. Here you participate against others who train at advanced levels.

Walking across the country

Your computer can also motivate you in another way. By going to www. discoverytrail.org, you can take a virtual walk on the American Discovery Trail, a 5,048-mile walk across America from Delaware to California.

Every time you walk, convert your steps into miles and see how far they take you along the trail. The page has links to all the sights you would see if you were actually on the trail. If you prefer, just eliminate the last two digits from the number of steps you take each day (so 10,000 steps becomes 100 miles). You will get across the country a lot faster that way than if you just convert your 10,000 steps into 4 or 5 miles. But what's the rush?

Just so you know, the trail can actually be walked or biked (or you can even ride a horse in some places). The eastern terminus is Cape Henlopen State Park in Delaware. The trail goes through Maryland, then West Virginia. It continues through Ohio where it splits in two directions. The northern route goes through Indiana, Illinois, Iowa, and Nebraska. The southern route takes you through Indiana, Illinois, Missouri, and Kansas. The routes join up again in Colorado and continue through Utah, Nevada, and California. The western terminus is at Point Reyes National Park in Marin County, California.

Adding Resistance Training to Your Program

Resistance training means exerting force against heavy weights. You can do it by using weights of different sizes that you buy or find in a fitness facility. Alternatively, you can use machines if you have access to them. The beauty of weights is that you can buy a set for your home and have them available whenever you need them. (Machines, on the other hand, are often too expensive and too large to purchase for home.)

Weightlifting is a form of anaerobic exercise. (See the sidebar earlier in this chapter if you're not sure what anaerobic exercise is.) It involves the movement of heavy weights, which can be moved only for brief periods of time. It results in significant muscle strengthening and increased endurance.

Doctors are always looking for drugs that can increase insulin sensitivity (see Chapter 10). But you need look no further than resistance training. Lifting weights has been shown in several studies to accomplish this goal. A September 2007 article in *Diabetes Care* written by a group of investigators from the CDC showed that muscle-strengthening activity significantly increased insulin sensitivity, thereby lowering the blood glucose and the hemoglobin A1c in 4,500 adults between the ages of 20 and 70.

Older adults (age 50 and above) who were given only eight weeks of flexibility and resistance training had substantial improvement in strength and flexibility while their glucose levels improved as well.

Weight training, which uses lighter weights, can be a form of aerobic exercise. Because the weights are light, they can be moved for prolonged periods of time. The result is improved cardiovascular fitness along with strengthening of muscles, tendons, ligaments, and bones. Weight training is an excellent way to protect and strengthen a joint that is beginning to develop some discomfort.

Doing resistance training with free weights

I recommend that you do seven different exercises with weights and one without weights at least two or three days a week if possible. Choose weights that permit you to do each exercise ten times in a row for three sets of ten with a rest in between. You should need only five to ten minutes to complete all eight, and the benefits will be huge. As you get stronger, increase the size of the weights. These exercises are the bicep curl, shoulder press, lateral raise, bent-over rowing, good mornings, flys, pullovers, and step-ups.

Figure 17-1 shows the bicep curl. To do this exercise:

1. **Hold the dumbbells along the sides of your body, palms facing forward.**
2. **Raise the dumbbells until your elbows are fully bent.**
3. **Slowly lower the dumbbells to the original position.**

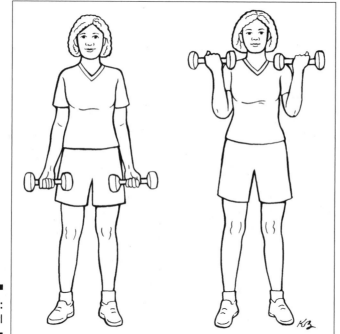

Figure 17-1:
Bicep curl

Figure 17-2 shows the shoulder press. To do this exercise:

1. **Hold the dumbbells with your palms facing each other and your elbows bent.**
2. **Raise the dumbbells over your head, turning your palms to face forward.**
3. **Lower the dumbbells to the original position.**

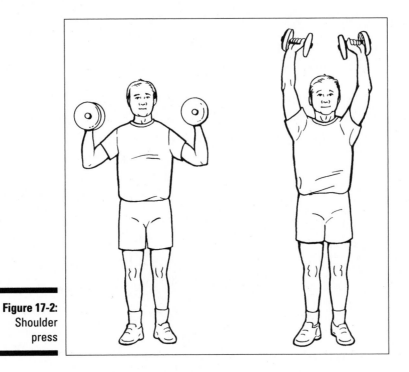

Figure 17-2:
Shoulder
press

Figure 17-3 shows the lateral raise. To do this exercise:

1. **Hold the dumbbells along the sides of your body, palms facing each other.**

2. **Lift the dumbbells out to the sides, palms facing the floor until they are above your head.**

3. **Lower the dumbbells down to your sides.**

Figure 17-4 shows bent-over rowing. To do this exercise:

1. **Hold a dumbbell in each hand, arms hanging down, legs straight, and back parallel to the floor.**

2. **Raise the dumbbells up to your chest.**

3. **Lower the dumbbells back to the floor.**

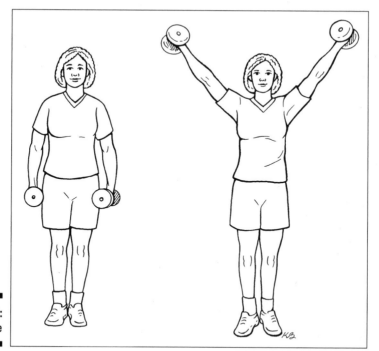

Figure 17-3:
Lateral raise

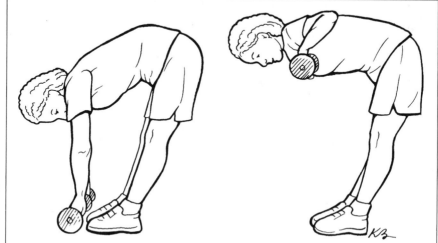

Figure 17-4:
Bent-over
rowing

Figure 17-5 shows good mornings. To do this exercise:

1. **Hold the ends of one dumbbell above your head, arms straight.**

2. **Lower the dumbbell forward as you bend your back parallel to the floor.**

3. **Raise the dumbbell to the original position.**

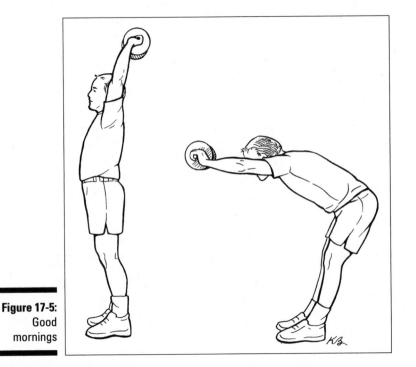

Figure 17-5:
Good
mornings

Figure 17-6 shows flys. To do this exercise:

1. **Lie on your back and hold the dumbbells out to each side at the shoulder.**

2. **Lift the dumbbells together until they are above your head.**

3. **Lower them to the sides again.**

Figure 17-7 shows pullovers. To do this exercise:

1. **Lie on your back holding one dumbbell with both hands straight up above your head.**

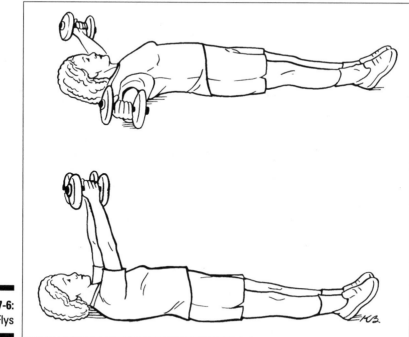

Figure 17-6:
Flys

2. **Lower the dumbbell with your arms straight to the floor behind your head.**

3. **Raise the dumbbell back above your head.**

Figure 17-8 shows step-ups. To do this exercise:

1. **Stand alongside the handrail at the bottom of a staircase.**

2. **With your feet flat and toes facing forward, put your right foot on the first step.**

3. **Straighten your right leg to lift up your left leg slowly until it reaches the first step.**

4. **Let your left foot land on the first step near your right.**

5. **Pause, then lower your left foot back to the floor.**

6. **Repeat ten times with your right foot on the first step and ten times with your left foot on the first step. Rest one to two minutes and do a second set.**

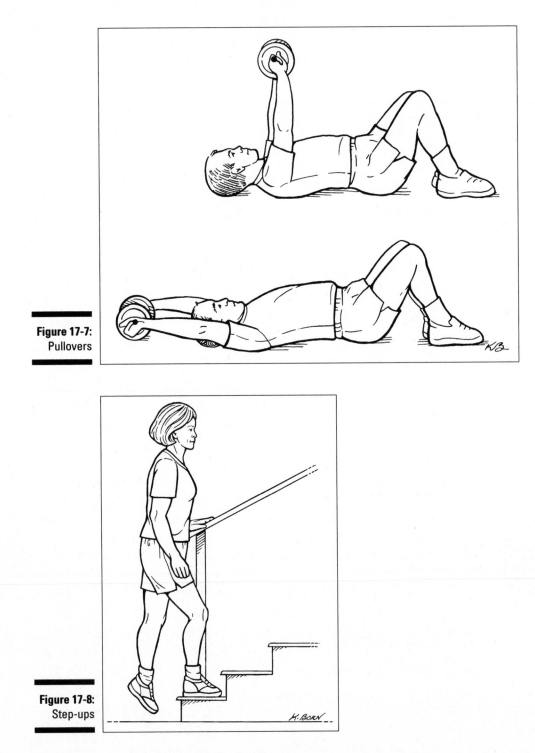

Figure 17-7:
Pullovers

Figure 17-8:
Step-ups

Older people in nursing homes who are given weights of just a few pounds have shown excellent return of strength to what appeared to be atrophied muscles. The benefits for you will be that much greater.

Weight training may be good for the days that you do not do your aerobic exercise, or you can add it for a few minutes after you finish your aerobic activity. Weight training is also good for working on a particular group of muscles that you feel is weak. Very often, these muscles are in the back. Weight-training exercises can isolate and strengthen each muscle.

If you do a lot of aerobic exercise that involves the legs, you may want to use upper body weight training only. I can tell you from personal experience that you not only feel a stronger upper body, but your ability to do your usual exercise is enhanced as well.

Doing resistance training using machines

All the exercises described in the previous section, with the exception of the step-ups, can be done using exercise machines. The advantage of machines is that the weights are part of the machine. If you become fatigued, you can just lower the weights under control.

I strongly recommend that you use an exercise trainer the first few times you use exercise machines. She can show you exactly how to use the machines properly, thereby avoiding injury. The trainer will also tell you how much weight to use at first and how much to increase the weight over time.

If you use a gym, you may find machines like the Cybex FT-450, which is a multipurpose machine that allows you to do every one of the exercises shown in this chapter. If you are looking for a home machine that allows all these exercises plus a lot more, the Body-Solid G41 Iso-Flex Home Gym simulates all free-weight exercises.

A good home machine like the Body Solid G41 may cost $2,000 or more. You may be better off joining an inexpensive health club for several months and using its machines until you are certain you will continue to use your machine at home. This way, if your early enthusiasm for resistance training turns to apathy, you won't be stuck owning a very expensive coat rack.

You can also find individual machines at fitness facilities to do each one of the exercises I show in this chapter. For example:

- ✔ Bicep curls can be done with Cybex's VR3 arm curl machine.
- ✔ Shoulder presses may be done with Cybex's VR3 overhead press machine.

- ✔ Lateral raises are done with Cybex's VR3 lateral raise machine.
- ✔ Bent-over rowing is done with Cybex's VR3 row machine.
- ✔ Good mornings are done with Cybex's lateral pull machine.
- ✔ Flys are done with Cybex's fly/rear delt machine.
- ✔ Pullovers are done with Cybex's VR3 pulldown machine.

These machines are designed so that the pattern of motion is correct. If you do the exercises with free weights without the help of a trainer, your motion may be wrong. With these machines, you can't get it wrong.

Are machines better than free weights or vice versa? The verdict is still out. If you use a fitness trainer to instruct you on the proper use of free weights, the two are probably the same.

Progressing with free weights or machines

How do you know how much weight to use at the beginning of your resistance training and how to progress with higher weights over time? If you are young (under 40), you should increase your performance over time. That means you continuously increase the resistance and the number of repetitions and sets.

If you are 40 or older, you need to be more careful of injury. You should keep the same weight if you experience a burning feeling in the exercised muscles for the last one to two minutes of your exercise. When you can do all your sets without a burning feeling, you are free to add more weight.

Chapter 18

Taking Medications or Supplements

In This Chapter

▶ Using medication to control prediabetes

▶ Studying the scientific research about various supplements

*B*ecause prediabetes is a relatively recent concept, doctors and researchers have not yet completely decided on using medications to treat it. In addition, prediabetes is generally not associated with the complications of diabetes — complications like those I discuss in Chapters 12, 13, and 14. As a result, prediabetes patients aren't usually prescribed the medications available to treat those complications.

However, a June 2009 article in *Population Health Management* reported that people with prediabetes have significantly more office visits for high blood pressure, kidney complications, and general medical conditions than people who don't have prediabetes. The article also reported that the annual cost of medical care for people with prediabetes is $25 billion. An intervention that can reverse medical problems such as high blood pressure and kidney complications — and save some of that money — is well worth discussing and utilizing.

There's an old joke about two ladies who go to a restaurant. One complains to the other that the food in this restaurant is really bad. The second one agrees and complains, "Not only that, but the portions are so small." As a grandfather taking a 2-year-old to a restaurant, I could add a second version: "Not only that, but there's no time to sit and eat it." Using medication for prediabetes is like that. Who wants to take medication at all? Not only that, but because prediabetes is a "predisease" and not a disease, you're not sure it's going to help anyway.

Nonetheless, if you make an honest effort at the lifestyle modifications I discuss in Chapters 15, 16, and 17 but are still struggling with prediabetes, medication is an obvious next step. In this chapter, I explain what your medication options are so you can discuss them with your doctor. In addition, I examine the scientific evidence regarding various supplements that are touted as helping people with prediabetes and diabetes.

Utilizing Medication

A number of medications are available right now to treat and perhaps reverse prediabetes. Useful medications should have the following characteristics:

✔ They should not cause weight gain.

✔ They should (we hope) cause weight loss.

✔ They should be easy to take.

✔ They should not have significant side effects that make the medications worse than the problems they are treating.

Several medications fulfill these criteria, and they are the subject of the next few pages.

 Your doctor must decide whether to provide you with these medications, but you need to be an informed consumer. You may even be the one who instigates the use of medication because many doctors are not yet fully tuned in to the concerns of prediabetes.

Starting with metformin

All drug treatment for prediabetes should probably start with metformin until and unless something better comes along. Since 1995, metformin has been approved in the United States for the treatment of diabetes.

While metformin is relatively new to the U.S. market, it has a longer history than the previous paragraph implies. A similar medication called phenformin had been banned in the United States because it caused a fatal complication called *lactic acidosis* (a condition where the blood becomes very acidic). As a result, the U.S. Food and Drug Administration (FDA) was reluctant to okay metformin until clinical studies proved it to be safe, even though it had been used for years in Europe with no problems.

How safe is metformin? In a July 2009 study published in *Critical Care Medicine,* people given an experimental overdose of metformin suffered no negative consequences. The only threat is to patients who already have multiple organ failure; if they are accidentally given an overdose of metformin, they may develop lactic acidosis and die. For everyone else, metformin is a safe drug.

Metformin has the following characteristics:

- ✔ It lowers your blood glucose mainly by reducing the production of glucose from your liver (what's called the *hepatic* glucose output).

- ✔ Used by itself, it does not cause *hypoglycemia* (a fall in blood glucose).

- ✔ Metformin may increase the sensitivity of your muscle cells to insulin and slow the uptake of glucose from your intestine.

- ✔ It must be taken with food because it causes gastrointestinal irritation, but this side effect declines with time.

- ✔ It's available in 500 mg, 850 mg, and 1,000 mg tablets.

- ✔ A relatively inexpensive generic form is available, which is just as good as any of the brand name forms. A liquid form is also available.

- ✔ The maximum daily dose is 2,500 mg taken in divided doses with each meal.

- ✔ It's often associated with weight loss, possibly from the gastrointestinal irritation or because it sometimes causes a loss of taste for food.

- ✔ It's not recommended when you have significant liver disease, kidney disease, or heart failure.

- ✔ It's usually stopped for a day or two before surgery or an x-ray study using a dye.

- ✔ It's not recommended for use in alcoholics.

- ✔ It's not recommended for use in pregnancy or by nursing mothers.

Metformin can be a very useful drug for prediabetes. Metformin has some positive effects on the blood fats, causing a decrease in triglycerides and LDL (bad) cholesterol and an increase in HDL (good) cholesterol (see Chapter 10).

What are the drawbacks? About 10 percent of patients fail to respond to metformin when it is first used, and the *secondary failure rate* (indicating how often the medication stops working after initially being successful) is 5 to 10 percent a year. Metformin also occasionally causes a decrease in the absorption of vitamin B_{12}, a vitamin that is important for the blood and the nervous system.

An excellent study of the effect of metformin in prediabetes was published in the journal *Canadian Family Physician* in April 2009. The study was a review and *meta-analysis,* meaning an examination of other acceptable papers on the subject. The article states that "Metformin decreases the rate of conversion from prediabetes to diabetes. This was true at higher dosage (850 mg twice daily) and lower dosage (250 mg twice or three times daily) [and] in people of varied ethnicity."

If diet and exercise have not reversed your prediabetes, discuss with your doctor the possibility of starting metformin at a low dose of 250 mg three times daily.

Moving to pioglitazone

Pioglitazone (brand name Actos) is a member of the class of drugs called thiazolidinediones (the glitazones). The first drug in this class was troglitazone, a very effective drug for lowering blood glucose. In 2000, troglitazone was taken off the market because of reports of liver failure leading to death in a small number of patients. The next thiazolidinedione was rosiglitazone (brand name Avandia), also very effective. However, some controversy exists as to whether rosiglitazone is associated with an increased rate of heart attacks. Studies have not confirmed this association, but I am wary of this drug.

Rosiglitazone has been shown to be effective in controlling and reversing prediabetes. A study presented at the meeting of the European Association for the Study of Diabetes in 2006 showed that rosiglitazone reduced the progression to diabetes by 62 percent among a group of 5,269 adults with prediabetes. Still, I would use this drug reluctantly. And because another thiazolidinedione is available that has *not* been associated with increased heart attacks, I prefer that drug: pioglitazone.

Pioglitazone was the third drug in this class to come to market. It has the following properties:

- ✔ Because it improves insulin resistance, this drug has its greatest effect on your blood glucose after you eat rather than after fasting (unlike metformin).

- ✔ By itself, pioglitazone does not cause hypoglycemia.

- ✔ Pioglitazone is *insulin sparing,* meaning your body does not have to make as much insulin to control your blood glucose.

- ✔ The drug is eliminated from your body almost entirely through your bowels, so no adjustment of the dose is needed if your kidneys are poorly functioning.

- ✔ So far, *secondary failure,* where the drug works initially but stops working later, does not seem to be a problem.

✔ The initial dose is 15 mg once a day with or without food.

✔ It restores fertility in some women who are infertile due to insulin resistance. In addition, it reduces estrogen levels in women taking estrogen and may result in making hormone-based contraception, such as oral contraceptive pills or depo-Provera, less effective.

✔ Pioglitazone has been shown to reduce LDL (bad) cholesterol in people with or without diabetes.

✔ It has been associated with increased osteoporosis in women.

✔ It does cause some weight gain due to water retention.

A study presented at the meeting of the American Diabetes Association in June 2008 showed that pioglitazone reduces the conversion of prediabetes to diabetes by 82 percent. That study involved starting with 30 mg daily and increasing the dose to 45 mg daily if the patient tolerates the drug. Within three months, pioglitazone significantly lowers the *fasting blood glucose* level (the amount of glucose in your blood after an overnight fast).

Because metformin causes weight loss and pioglitazone causes weight gain, I would still use metformin as the drug of first choice for the treatment of prediabetes.

Injecting insulin

Recent evidence suggests that using insulin very early in the development of type 2 diabetes reverses the disease and results in much longer remission rates than using oral agents such as metformin and pioglitazone. A May 2008 study published in *The Lancet* showed that 98 percent of patients recently diagnosed with type 2 diabetes could achieve control of their blood glucose by using insulin. Also, when their normal blood glucose levels were maintained for two weeks, they could stop taking the insulin. Fifty percent of the people in this study who used insulin remained in remission after one year. (By comparison, the remission rate after a year for people taking pills was only 26 percent.)

But you don't have type 2 diabetes yet, so what does this information have to do with your situation? Some researchers have suggested that the short-term use of insulin will work even better in patients with prediabetes than in patients newly diagnosed with type 2 diabetes. After all, in prediabetes, your blood glucose levels haven't been abnormal for very long and aren't as far off track as in someone with type 2 diabetes. A study is now underway using *insulin glargine,* a long-acting type of insulin, to determine if early use will reverse prediabetes and result in long-term remission. A small initial study showed that this approach is feasible.

The potential problems of using insulin in prediabetes include hypoglycemia, weight gain, the unpredictability of long-acting insulin, and the need for injections. Ask your doctor about this possible treatment because much more will be known about it in the near future.

Considering GLP-1

This new class of drugs has a different mechanism from any of the previous classes of oral agents. A hormone called *glucagon-like peptide-1* (GLP-1), which is made in the small intestine, has a number of positive effects for people with diabetes:

- ✔ It slows the movement of food in the intestine, thus slowing the absorption of glucose.
- ✔ It reduces the production of glucagon from the pancreas. Glucagon raises the blood glucose.
- ✔ It lowers the hemoglobin A1c (see Chapter 10) and the blood glucose.
- ✔ It increases insulin levels.
- ✔ It does not cause hypoglycemia when used by itself.
- ✔ It decreases food intake, which leads to weight loss.
- ✔ It normalizes the blood glucose in many patients.

The problem with naturally occurring GLP-1 is that it is rapidly broken down by an enzyme called *DPP-4*. Therefore, under usual circumstances, GLP-1 is not around long enough to have these effects in a major way.

Exenatide (brand name Byetta) is a powerful form of GLP-1 that lasts for several hours. It is injected within an hour before breakfast and supper. It comes in pens containing either 5 or 10 micrograms per dose. It can sometimes cause substantial weight loss and is associated with nausea. On rare occasions, it can't be used because the nausea is so severe.

Several longer-acting versions of exenatide will soon be available. One will require only a single shot daily. Another will require taking only one shot a week. Studies have shown that these versions control glucose even better than twice-daily exenatide. These drugs may play a large role in the treatment of prediabetes in the future.

Looking at DPP-4 inhibitors

In the previous section, I point out that natural GLP-1 in the body is limited by its rapid breakdown by an enzyme called *DPP-4*. The action of natural

GLP-1 can be prolonged if you take a substance that blocks the action of the enzyme. Scientists have been able to make several such drugs called *DPP-4 inhibitors*. Three DPP-4 inhibitors have been created, only one of which is currently available to patients.

Sitagliptin

This drug has the brand name Januvia and comes in 25, 50, and 100 mg versions. The usual dose is 100 mg daily. Because sitagliptin is excreted by the kidneys, people with kidney disease must take lower doses. It can cause stomach discomfort.

The problem with sitagliptin is that it lowers your *hemoglobin A1c* (an indicator of your blood glucose level for the past three months) less than 1 percent. In addition, it does not result in weight loss, which I believe is the major advantage of GLP-1. However, sitagliptin could be an ideal drug for some people because its milder effect may be just what is needed. So far, no major study of sitagliptin use for prediabetes has been done.

Vildagliptin and saxagliptin

Vildagliptin (brand name Galvus) and saxagliptin (brand name Onglyza) are very similar to sitagliptin in their effects. The FDA has not yet authorized their sale in the United States, but vildagliptin is authorized for use within the European Union.

Researching Supplement Claims

Any time you have a disease that affects millions of people, you are bound to hear claims that the absence of a certain micronutrient is the cause of the disease. Therefore, you hear claims that a certain supplement can cure the disease. Because prediabetes affects so many people, you'll likely hear a huge number of claims about a wide variety of supplements that can benefit your blood glucose levels and help reduce your risk for associated conditions, such as heart disease. Are any of them true? In this section, I tell you what scientific evidence exists for any of these claims.

Chromium

You can find articles singing the praises of chromium for controlling the symptoms of diabetes in all kinds of magazines and newspapers, and on the Internet. Logically, if chromium works for diabetes, it should work even better for prediabetes. Should you take supplements of chromium?

The strongest case for chromium comes from a study of people with type 2 diabetes in China. They were given high doses of chromium and were found to improve their hemoglobin A1c, blood glucose, and cholesterol while reducing the amount of insulin they had to take. However, these people were chromium deficient in the first place. People in the United States and other countries where the diet is sufficient in chromium do not have this deficiency and do not show improvement in glucose tolerance when they take chromium. In addition, chromium is present in such small amounts normally that it is hard to measure even in people without chromium deficiency.

The exact amount of chromium you need in your diet is uncertain, but estimates indicate 15 to 50 micrograms daily. People who take much more than that amount tend to accumulate the chromium in their livers, where it can be toxic. Some studies suggest that chromium in high doses can cause cancer.

For now, the evidence does not support the use of chromium in prediabetes or diabetes except for people who are known to be chromium deficient.

Aspirin

People who take the *sulfonylurea drugs* (a class of drugs that lowers blood glucose by stimulating more insulin production) for diabetes sometimes have a greater drop in blood glucose when they take aspirin. This happens because aspirin competes with the other drug for binding sites on the proteins that carry sulfonylureas in the blood. When they're bound to protein, the sulfonylureas are not active; when they're free, they are. Aspirin knocks the sulfonylureas off so that they're free. As a result, aspirin has been recommended as a drug to lower blood glucose.

By itself, aspirin has little effect on blood glucose. And its effect with sulfonylureas is so inconsistent that it can't be reliably depended upon to lower your blood glucose. Finally, because people with prediabetes do not take sulfonylureas, aspirin can't be expected to have any effect for them.

Cinnamon

A number of articles in the medical literature since 2001 have suggested that cinnamon lowers the blood glucose in type 2 diabetes and improves fat levels as well. To verify these claims, a study called a *meta-analysis* was done and published in *Diabetes Care* in January 2008. In a *meta-analysis,* all studies that are *randomized* (so the subjects don't know if they are getting the drug or a placebo) are analyzed to see if they confirm the hypothesis. In this case, none of the five studies analyzed showed that cinnamon had a positive effect either on blood glucose or blood fats. You may have noticed the same thing if you were taking a daily dose of a teaspoon of cinnamon. You can cease and desist! Taking cinnamon doesn't help in diabetes and won't help in prediabetes.

Pancreas Formula

Pancreas Formula is sold on the Internet as a mixture of herbs, vitamins, and minerals that help diabetes and prediabetes. No clinical or experimental evidence shows that pancreas formula does anything of value in the human body. The claims that are made for this "treatment" are not supported by factual evidence.

Fat Burner

You may hear and read a lot of advertising for the Fat Burner product in reputable newspapers and on reputable radio stations. The advertisements claim that you can "burn fat without diet or exercise," and they even throw in, ABSOLUTELY FREE, a bottle of Spirulina to enhance your Fat Burner weight control program. If you believe you can burn fat by simply taking a pill, I have a bridge I would like to sell you, *cheap.* In order to burn fat, you must exercise and stop consuming large amounts of fats, carbohydrates, or other sources of calories.

Ki-Sweet

The literature for Ki-Sweet offers another lesson in being skeptical. The creators of this "miracle" sweetener claim that it has a "special designation from the American Diabetes Association." The ADA denies the claim, but how many people will buy something when they see ADA approval and not bother to see whether it's true? No evidence exists that Ki-Sweet, made by squeezing the juice of the kiwi fruit, has any advantages over other sweeteners either in diabetes or prediabetes.

Gymnema sylvestre

Gymnema sylvestre is a plant found in India and Africa that is promoted as a glucose-lowering agent as part of an alternative medical treatment called *Ayurvedic medicine.* Gymnema sylvestre has never been tested in a controlled study in humans. One statement in its advertising is, "For most people, blood sugar lowers to normal levels." No evidence exists that this is the case.

Vitamin supplements

In Chapter 10, I discuss vitamins: what they do, how you get them, and how they can be measured to see whether you have a deficiency. The question here is whether a lack of a certain vitamin makes you more likely to develop prediabetes and whether taking one or many vitamins is necessary for your health.

Volumes have been written by well-meaning people proclaiming the need for vitamin supplements. Unfortunately, the proof they offer is an anecdote here and an anecdote there. You never find a study in a well-known medical journal that compares two groups, one that gets the supplement and one that doesn't, with no one knowing which is which, including the doctors. That is known as a *double-blind study* (because both the participants and doctors are "blind" regarding who is getting the supplement), and it's the gold standard for determining how effective a supplement or medication really is. Data is collected before, during, and at the end of the study to see who improves and who does not. Only at the end do the doctors and participants find out who got the real stuff and who got the placebo. If the supplement or medicine really makes a difference, a significant number of people who took it should see much greater improvement than those who didn't.

Double-blind studies have not shown that vitamin supplements are helpful to most people. Instead, they have shown that a healthy person who eats a balanced and varied diet (like the one I describe in Chapter 16) normally obtains enough vitamins and minerals to meet his needs. People who don't eat a balanced diet or who have special needs may need to take a vitamin and mineral supplement. People with special needs would include the elderly (especially those who live at home alone), women during pregnancy and lactation, and people who are on diets to lose weight. Since you, dear reader, are going to significantly improve your diet on my advice, you don't need a vitamin supplement. If you don't improve your diet, you may need one — but check with your doctor.

Recent studies have shown that increased blood levels of *homocysteine,* an amino acid, are high in people with cardiovascular disease. Because deficiencies of folic acid (vitamin B_9), pyridoxine (vitamin B_6), and cyanocobalamin (vitamin B_{12}) lead to high homocysteine levels, the studies recommended taking those vitamins to prevent heart disease. However, studies of supplementation have not shown benefits, and some studies have actually shown increased risks of heart disease for people who take supplements.

Biotin (vitamin B_7) is another vitamin that has been touted as a useful supplement in prediabetes. It is said to be essential for the manufacture of insulin and has insulin-like properties. B_7 helps to maintain a steady glucose level in the blood. However, deficiency is extremely rare because you need very little, and what you need is produced by intestinal bacteria. No proof exists that supplementation of biotin is necessary.

Save your money! Don't buy vitamins and minerals unless you have a special need or you have tests done that prove you are vitamin deficient.

Antioxidant supplements

Antioxidants are substances that slow or prevent the oxidation of other substances. Oxidation produces *free radicals,* substances that damage or kill cells. Antioxidants are widely used in dietary supplements with the hope of maintaining health and preventing heart disease, cancer, and some of the complications of high blood glucose.

Large clinical trials have not verified the benefits of antioxidant supplements, and some clinical trials have shown potential harm from antioxidants. For example, there is an increased risk of lung cancer when beta-carotene is given to smokers. There is an increased risk of heart failure and possibly death when high doses of vitamin E are taken.

Instead of taking an antioxidant supplement, I highly recommend consuming food sources of antioxidants: fruits, vegetables, whole grains, and vegetable oils.

Soy protein

In an article in *The New England Journal of Medicine* in 1995, this supplement was declared to reduce total cholesterol, LDL (bad) cholesterol, and triglycerides. The article was based on a study paid for by DuPont, which makes soy protein. As a result, the FDA allowed DuPont to make a health claim about soy protein, that it "may reduce the risk of heart disease."

In January 2006, the American Heart Association (AHA) published a study in the journal *Circulation* that reviewed the 1995 study, as well as more recent studies. The 2006 article denied the claim that soy protein is good for the heart, as well as claims that soy protein reduces hot flashes in menopausal women and prevents cancer of the breast, uterus, and prostate. The AHA did not recommend soy protein supplements.

However, the AHA article did indicate that soy products like soy nuts and tofu should be beneficial to health because they contain a high concentration of polyunsaturated fats, fiber, vitamins, and minerals. If soy protein replaces animal proteins that contain saturated fats and cholesterol, its use in your diet should be beneficial.

Phytochemicals

Phytochemicals are substances like flavonoids and sulphur-containing compounds that help to explain the benefits of fruits and vegetables in reducing coronary heart disease. Many phytochemicals are found in fruits and vegetables, but we don't know which ones are beneficial. No study has shown that a specific phytochemical is beneficial. Therefore, I do not recommended taking phytochemicals as supplements. Instead, you should try to eat a diet that includes the amounts of fruits and vegetables recommended in the U.S. Government Food Pyramid (see Chapter 16).

Processing foods removes their phytochemicals — one of many reasons to avoid processed food in favor of unprocessed food.

Fish oil supplements

Eating more fish, especially oily fish, has been associated with lower incidences of heart disease. Studies of people around the Mediterranean Sea who eat lots of oily fish show the benefits of this food. The current recommendation is to eat oily fish at least twice a week. Here are the fish that contain the highest levels of fish oil:

- Mackerel
- Lake trout
- Herring
- Sardines
- Albacore tuna
- Salmon

Mackerel and albacore tuna may contain excessive amounts of mercury so you should be careful about how much you consume of these fish. The recommendation is three servings or less per month.

In place of oily fish, which contains omega-3 fatty acids, supplements of omega-3 fish oils may be beneficial. Two omega-3 fatty acids are found in fish oil: docosahexaenoic acid (DHA) and eicosapentaenoic acid (EPA). A number of benefits are associated with fish oil supplements. These include:

- Decreased pain from inflammation
- Reduction in cardiovascular disease
- Reduction in blood pressure
- Reduction in stroke and heart attack

✔ Improved brain function

✔ Reduction in depression and psychosis

✔ Decrease in cancer of the breast, colon, and prostate

Alpha-linolenic acid is another omega-3 fatty acid that is found in English walnuts and vegetable oils, including canola oil, soybean oil, flaxseed/oil, linseed oil, and olive oil. The benefits of alpha-linolenic acid have not been proved as strongly as the omega-3s in fish. It is actually converted into the fish oil omega-3s but only to a limited extent in the body.

The omega-3 fatty acids do not seem to have any effect on blood glucose.

Alpha-lipoic acid and racemic lipoic acid

These two different structural forms of the same compound have been recommended for controlling blood glucose and improving insulin function. This action has been shown only in cell cultures, however, and not in animals or people. In fact, alpha-lipoic acid makes type 1 diabetes worse in rats.

These two acids are found in almost all foods but in very tiny amounts. Alpha-lipoic acid is also made by the body so deficiencies are very unlikely.

Alpha-lipoic acid is also an antioxidant, and you may read claims that it prevents or treats many age-related diseases like diabetes, Parkinson's disease, and Alzheimer's disease. No studies have been done to prove these claims one way or the other. We don't know how much dosage would be used for combating any disease, and I do not recommend supplementation with alpha-lipoic acid until more research is done.

Pycnogenol

Pycnogenol is an extract from the bark of the French maritime pine. It consists of a blend of compounds with antioxidant properties. Some people claim that Pycnogenol lowers blood glucose levels, but this claim has not been confirmed by research. Other claims about Pycnogenol include that it can:

✔ Improve asthma

✔ Improve *chronic venous insufficiency,* a condition where the legs are swollen because blood pools in the lower body

✔ Protect cells (because of its antioxidant properties)

✔ Improve concentration in attention deficit hyperactivity disorder

- ✔ Reduce pain during menstruation
- ✔ Reduce swelling due to water retention
- ✔ Reduce plaque formation in the mouth
- ✔ Reduce blood pressure
- ✔ Reduce LDL (bad) cholesterol and increase HDL (good) cholesterol
- ✔ Improve male infertility
- ✔ Reduce the frequency and severity of migraine headaches
- ✔ Prevent blood clots during long airplane rides
- ✔ Slow the progression of diabetic eye disease
- ✔ Reduce redness caused by sunburn

You would think from this list that Pycnogenol is a wonder drug, but none of the claims have been proved. The drug is not recommended as treatment for prediabetes or anything else.

Chapter 19

Considering Bariatric Surgery

Surgery to reverse prediabetes, which is really synonymous with surgery for obesity, may seem like an overreaction, especially because prediabetes often involves few if any symptoms. But the truth is that if an overweight patient can't get his or her weight under control, that person is in for a lot of potential misery. When you add up the future medical expenses and time lost from work because of illness, and you also consider the poor quality (and shortened quantity) of life that person faces, surgery doesn't seem so drastic.

The annual number of weight loss surgery operations in the United States is about 200,000. Consider that 100 million or more Americans are obese (meaning their body mass index is 30 or greater — see Chapter 6), and you can bet that in the next few years the number of surgeries is going to grow.

In this chapter, I explain your weight loss surgery options. I list the criteria for deciding whether to even consider it, help you figure out which type of weight loss surgery is the one for you, show how to decide on a surgeon, and discuss what happens after surgery.

As he lay on his death bed, the bon vivant Richard Milnes observed, "My exit is the result of too many entrees." If you have surgery for obesity, you will have to significantly reduce the number of entrees that you eat, but in return your exit will take place a lot later.

Deciding That Diet and Exercise Are Not Enough

A number of benefits are associated with weight loss surgery, but not everyone who suffers from sickness associated with obesity is a candidate.

Realizing the possible benefits of surgery

Weight loss surgery reverses or greatly improves a number of conditions that are a consequence of obesity. The benefits may include:

- Reversal of prediabetes to normal glucose metabolism
- Reversal of diabetes 80 percent of the time so that medication is not needed
- Reversal of high blood pressure to normal
- Elimination of gastrointestinal abnormalities like acid reflux and heartburn
- Elimination of sleep apnea
- Improvement in sexual quality of life and abnormalities in reproduction hormones in men
- Great improvement in shortness of breath and mobility
- Improvement or elimination of back pain, joint pain, and arthritis
- Reversal of infertility in women
- Improved quality of life

Meeting the criteria for surgery

A number of guidelines determine whether you meet the criteria to have surgery for obesity. Here are some of the more important ones:

- You are at high risk for a disease like diabetes, heart attack, or stroke.
- You have a genetic condition that causes obesity.
- You have a body mass index greater than 40 (see Chapter 6).

  ✔ You have a body mass index greater than 35 plus significant disease like high blood pressure, heart disease, sleep apnea, or diabetes.

  ✔ You are at least 100 pounds overweight or 100 percent larger than your ideal weight, which is considered *morbid obesity.*

  ✔ You are between the ages of 18 and 64.

  ✔ You have no known metabolic or endocrine cause for your morbid obesity.

  ✔ You are motivated and able to participate in long-term follow up.

  ✔ You have tried dieting, medication, and exercise without success.

If you meet several of these criteria, you are a candidate for surgery.

Picking the Right Kind of Surgery

The two major choices for weight loss surgery are gastric bypass and adjustable gastric banding. I explain each in this section. In either case, the surgery should be done using a *laparoscope,* a small tube that enters the abdomen, requiring only a small opening. Rarely, a patient will not be able to have the surgery with a laparoscope but will require a large incision instead. Recovery after a large incision is more difficult.

Focusing on gastric bypass

Gastric bypass is a much more invasive and extensive surgery than gastric banding. It accounts for 80 percent of the weight loss surgeries in the United States. Here, I discuss how the surgery is done, its potential complications, and typical results.

How the surgery is done

Figure 19-1 shows the appearance of your stomach and intestines after gastric bypass surgery. The operation is usually done with a *laparoscope,* a tube that is manipulated remotely through four or five small incisions to minimize surgical trauma. A small pouch of your stomach, which is attached to the *esophagus* (the tube between your mouth and stomach), is separated from the rest of the stomach. The pouch is about the size of a golf ball. The pouch is made so small because it will stretch after surgery and the surgeon wants the final size to be small after stretching. The part of the stomach to which the pouch was previously attached is closed.

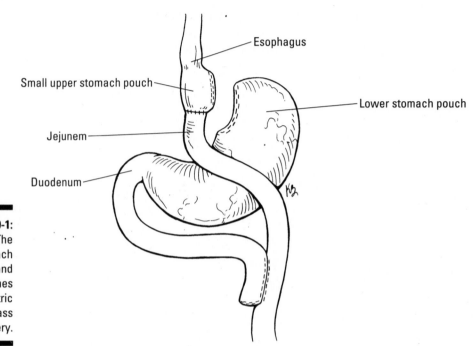

Figure 19-1:
The stomach and intestines after gastric bypass surgery.

Esophagus

Small upper stomach pouch

Lower stomach pouch

Jejunem

Duodenum

Your small intestine, which connects the stomach with the large intestine, is cut. The part of the small intestine that connects at the other end to the large intestine is connected to the upper stomach pouch. Now there is a continuous path for food from your mouth, through the esophagus, into the pouch, into the shortened small intestine, and into the large intestine.

At this point, the large portion of your stomach remains attached to the upper, bypassed small intestine (usually about 1.5 to 5 feet of a total length of 20 feet), which is still open at its end. That open end is attached to the side of your small intestine that connects the small pouch to the large intestine. The result is that gastric digestive juices from your stomach and bypassed small intestine can mix with the food you eat to aid digestion. Why is the lower stomach left there instead of being removed altogether? This way, it can be reattached if you need the operation reversed. Also, removing it would greatly prolong the surgery and increase possible complications.

After having the surgery, you feel full after eating very small quantities of food. In addition, your shortened intestine does not fully absorb vitamins and minerals.

Potential complications of gastric bypass

The most serious complication of any surgery, of course, is death. The risk of dying during bypass surgery is less than 1 percent, especially in the hands of an experienced surgeon.

Within the first 30 days after surgery, any of the following may occur:

- There may be a leak at one of the connections, which could cause severe inflammation and infection.

- Your bowels can become obstructed.

- You may experience nausea, vomiting, and diarrhea as you adjust to the new limitations on your stomach and digestive system.

- Your surgical wound may cause pain.

- Hemorrhage may occur.

- If you have sleep apnea, you may become sleep-deprived. That's because you can't use the machine that usually allows you to sleep; doing so could cause a rupture of the surgical connection.

- A blood clot may form that travels into your lungs (*pulmonary embolism*).

Over the long term, you deal with further complications:

- The procedure is expensive, costing $25,000 or more, which some insurance plans will not pay.

- Recovery can take up to three months, during which time you may be out of work.

- You have to limit your food choices for the rest of your life because the wrong food can cause blockage or *dumping syndrome,* a feeling of abdominal cramps and nausea when undigested food is "dumped" into your small intestine too rapidly. Other symptoms are dizziness, rapid heart rate, sweating, weakness, and fatigue. The main foods that cause this problem are high carbohydrate foods like cookies and donuts — foods you shouldn't be eating anyway.

- For best results, you have to do an hour of exercise daily, which may be a burden if you aren't used to doing exercise.

- The surgery is permanent and can't be adjusted without further surgery.

- Vitamin and mineral deficiencies can result from malabsorption, especially of several B vitamins, vitamin D, iron, and calcium. Malabsorption of iron can cause anemia.

- It is possible to out-eat the bypass and gain weight or not lose much weight.

Results of bypass surgery

Most studies show that gastric bypass patients lose 60 to 70 percent of their excess weight. A January 2008 study in the journal *Surgery* also showed that gastric bypass surgery also reduced patients' ten-year risk of a heart attack by more than 50 percent.

What about diabetes? A meta-analysis study published in *The American Journal of Medicine* in March 2009 looked at 621 different studies of gastric bypass and determined that the surgery normalized or improved diabetes in 90 percent of cases. The study also showed that gastric bypass is considerably more successful than adjustable gastric banding (which I discuss in the next section). Eighty percent of gastric bypass patients had total resolution of diabetes, while 57 percent of gastric banding patients achieved that result. (However, a November 2007 study in the *Journal of the American College of Surgeons* looked at 282 patients who had bariatric surgery and determined there was no difference between gastric bypass and gastric banding in the rate of resolution of diabetes.)

Because gastric bypass is so successful at reversing diabetes, it likely will be even more successful at preventing prediabetes from becoming diabetes and returning patients to a normal metabolism. The studies have not yet been published, but that result is fairly certain.

Opting for adjustable gastric banding

The second major weight loss operation is *adjustable gastric banding*. Though not done as often as gastric bypass in the United States, this surgery is much more popular in the rest of the world. Figure 19-2 shows the stomach after adjustable gastric banding.

How the surgery is done

Like gastric bypass, this surgery is done with a *laparoscope,* a tube that is manipulated remotely through four or five small incisions to minimize surgical trauma. The surgeon straps an inflatable silicone cuff around your stomach, dividing the stomach into a tiny upper pouch with a restricted opening to the much larger lower pouch. The cuff can be loosened or tightened using a syringe to adjust the amount of saline solution in a port implanted under your skin.

The tiny stomach pouch fills very quickly and empties very slowly so you feel full after eating very little. If you overeat, food backs up into your esophagus, which feels very unpleasant. You learn to eat very little at a time and to chew your food very thoroughly.

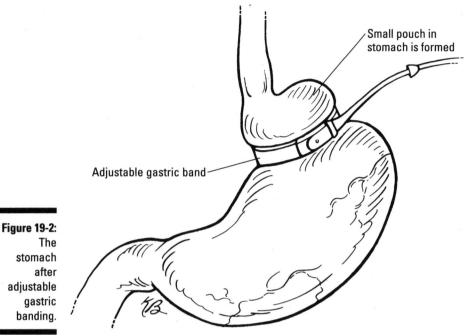

Small pouch in
stomach is formed

Adjustable gastric band

Figure 19-2:
The
stomach
after
adjustable
gastric
banding.

Advantages of gastric banding

Gastric banding is much less invasive and requires much less surgery than
gastric bypass. Here are some of the advantages compared to gastric bypass:

- ✔ The hospital stay is shorter.
- ✔ The death rate is extremely low.
- ✔ You don't become anemic due to malabsorption of iron.
- ✔ You don't experience dumping syndrome, which I describe in the section on gastric bypass.
- ✔ You don't struggle with malabsorption of vitamins and minerals (because your intestines aren't involved in the surgery).

Potential complications of adjustable gastric banding

Because it is the least invasive of the operations for weight loss, adjustable
gastric banding has few problems at the time of surgery. In the short term
after surgery, you may experience infection at the site of the syringe that is
used to adjust the gastric band.

Here are some of the longer term complications you could experience:

- ✔ Your stomach may perforate.
- ✔ A hernia may occur at the incision site.
- ✔ The opening to the larger stomach pouch may narrow or close.
- ✔ The gastric band can slip.
- ✔ The tube from the port under your skin can leak or break.
- ✔ The gastric band can erode into your stomach.
- ✔ Surgery may be needed to revise the position of the band or reverse the operation.

Results of adjustable gastric banding

People who have adjustable gastric banding lose 40 to 55 percent of their excess weight by two years after surgery. They improve the various conditions associated with obesity like prediabetes, diabetes, high blood pressure, and heart disease, but not as much as patients who have the gastric bypass operation. For example, diabetes returns to normal glucose metabolism in 80 percent of patients who have gastric bypass but only 57 percent who have adjustable gastric banding.

Habits of successful surgery patients

Successful weight loss surgery patients seem to have certain habits in common. To increase your chances for success after either gastric bypass or gastric banding, here's what you need to do:

- ✔ Eat three balanced meals and two snacks daily.
- ✔ Drink water but no carbonated beverages.
- ✔ If you've had gastric bypass, take daily multiple vitamins, calcium, and iron.
- ✔ Sleep at least seven hours per night.
- ✔ Exercise at least four times per week for at least 40 minutes each time.
- ✔ Take personal responsibility for following your program.

Weighing pros and cons of each

Which surgery (if either) is right for you? That's a question that only you and your doctor can answer after spending a great deal of time considering your individual circumstances. But I do suggest that you keep the following facts in mind as you weigh pros and cons:

- ✔ Adjustable gastric banding is a more benign surgery with fewer complications.

- ✔ However, adjustable gastric banding requires more frequent reoperation than gastric bypass.

- ✔ Gastric bypass leads to greater weight loss with more significant reversal of the complications of obesity.

For my patients, I often recommend gastric bypass over adjustable gastric banding as the surgery of choice because the results are more dramatic. But again, only you and your doctor have the complete information in order to make your decision.

Although it is not usually emphasized, several years of freedom from diabetes or complete control of the blood glucose can have a lasting impact, as shown by the two major studies of diabetic control: the Diabetes Control and Complications Trial for type 1 diabetes and the United Kingdom Prospective Diabetes Study for type 2 diabetes. The studies showed a *legacy effect:* Ten years after the surgery, even patients who had lost their formerly tight control over their weight and their diabetes still showed reduced risk for heart attacks and other causes of death. Even if you have only a few years of reduced weight, you will have benefits.

Choosing the Right Surgeon

The right surgeon can make the difference between a complication-free surgery and smooth recovery (with positive results) and a difficult surgery filled with complications followed by inadequate weight loss (and possibly even a second operation). In this section, I show you how to go about finding the right surgeon.

Figuring out your options

Often your doctor (your primary care physician or endocrinologist) will choose the surgeon you're going to work with. You'll likely agree to that choice, assuming that your doctor has your best interests at heart. Usually, your doctor does have your best interests at heart, so this is a pretty good method for picking a surgeon. However, sometimes other factors determine the doctor's choice. The surgeon may be a golfing buddy or a colleague with whom your doctor has been working for years. Or your doctor may want to keep your case within the confines of a particular hospital.

Sometimes your insurance company trumps your doctor's choice. Insurance companies often mandate that you can only go to certain surgeons to have this surgery performed.

What if your doctor or your insurance company doesn't pick a surgeon for you? Who do you ask for suggestions? You could ask a friend or colleague who has had weight-loss surgery, but I strongly advise doing your own research after getting a name or two to consider.

The three most important criteria for a surgeon are experience, experience and experience. Surgeons who do weight loss operations once a month are not experienced. Surgeons who do this type of operation several times a week are experienced.

Several studies have shown that the lowest risk of complications and the most successful surgical result come from a surgical team that has done at least 125 previous operations. You may say, "That's a Catch-22! How is a surgeon supposed to get 125 operations under his belt if no one will use him because he has only done 20 operations?" Let someone else answer that question. You use only the most experienced surgeon you can find.

Perhaps the best way to find a surgeon to do your weight loss surgery is by going to the Web site of the Surgical Review Corporation. This is an independent group that was created by the American Society for Metabolic and Bariatric Surgery. The purpose was to designate surgical programs that meet strict standards for weight loss surgery. You can find the Surgical Review Corporation at www.surgicalreview.org/index.aspx.

The Surgical Review Corporation was established to assess and improve the efficacy, efficiency, and safety of bariatric surgery. To accomplish this, here's what the organization does:

- Formulates and establishes guidelines and criteria for assessing bariatric surgical practices

- Evaluates and investigates applicants to ensure they meet established standards for recognition as a Bariatric Surgery Center of Excellence

- Collects, analyzes, and disseminates data in compliance with applicable privacy limitations and other applicable laws and regulations

As I write these words (in mid-2009), 381 U.S. facilities are recognized as Bariatric Surgery Centers of Excellence and 635 surgeons are recognized as highly qualified to perform the surgery.

At the Surgical Review Corporation Web site, click on "Locate a Center of Excellence." When a large map appears, click on your state. For example, I clicked on California and was presented with a list of 37 cities that have at least one such center with numerous physicians who can perform the surgery. (In contrast, Hawaii had no listings at the time of this writing.)

The fact that a center is not on the list does not mean that it has failed a test for quality. Some very fine centers choose not to be evaluated by the Surgical Review Corporation, especially academic medical centers.

Asking the right questions

So you have settled on a medical center to have the surgery, and you think you know the surgeon you want to do it. Now you have to evaluate the surgeon. This is not a one-time sale, where you will never see the salesperson again. You are going to become very intimate with this doctor, and you want to be sure it's the right match. Here are the questions you should ask and the answers you want to get:

- ✔ **Are you board-certified in general surgery?** (Currently there is no separate board certification in gastrointestinal surgery.) Answer: Yes

- ✔ **Are you affiliated with the American Society for Bariatric Surgery?** Answer: Yes.

- ✔ **Have you done at least 125 surgeries for weight loss?** Answer: Yes.

- ✔ **What is your success rate?** Answer: 80 to 90 percent of patients lose at least 50 to 60 percent of excess weight.

- ✔ **Do you use laparoscopy-assisted surgical methods?** Answer: Yes.

- ✔ **What is your rate of complications?** Answer: Under 10 percent.

- ✔ **What post-operative support do you offer?** Answer: Lifelong follow-up is included.

- ✔ **Will you quickly answer e-mail questions?** Answer: Yes.

- ✔ **Do you have dietitians or nutritionists on the staff?** Answer: Yes.

Here are some other things you can find out without asking the doctor directly:

- ✔ **Has the doctor been disciplined for any infractions?** You can learn this information by contacting the state medical licensing organization.

- ✔ **Does the doctor look at you when he talks to and examines you?**

- ✔ **Does the doctor listen to you and respond to your questions?**

> ✔ **Do you feel you are getting enough time?** You definitely don't want to be rushed.
>
> ✔ **Is the doctor's staff helpful and happy?** If so, that suggests they feel good about working for this caregiver.
>
> ✔ **Does the doctor's office appear clean and well-maintained?**
>
> ✔ **Do other patients in the office appear happy to be there?**

Pinpointing the costs you have to cover

Weight loss surgery currently costs about $25,000, which includes:

> ✔ Hospital fees
>
> ✔ Surgeon fees
>
> ✔ Anesthesia fees
>
> ✔ Lab and x-ray fees
>
> ✔ Miscellaneous fees

You can pay these fees in a number of ways. Of course, if your health insurance pays for the surgery, you're off the hook financially. But if insurance refuses to pay (which you should know long before surgery), you may have to finance the surgery with a loan.

Preparing for Surgery

Any kind of surgery is more successful if you can prepare for it. Luckily, because weight loss surgery is elective, you can schedule it to allow enough time to get yourself ready. Here's how.

Getting ready mentally and physically

Much needs to be done before you get on the table and turn your stomach into a small cup. Weight loss surgery results in a lifelong change in your lifestyle, and you need to be prepared.

It's very helpful if you can talk to people who have had the surgery to find out what to expect. Your experience will probably not be the same, but there will be some similarities.

Start a journal so you can record your progress, your setbacks, and your feelings. The journal will provide valuable information that you can look back on as you go through the changes involved in getting rid of half of you.

 Make sure you enlist your family. Get them to go with you to the dietitian, who will suggest what and how you can eat after the surgery. Also take them along to meetings where you learn about the consequences of your surgery. Your weight loss will have a great effect on your family dynamics, so make sure your family members are informed.

Start your physical preparation months before the actual surgery. Here are some of the things you should do:

✔ Develop an exercise and fitness plan several months before the surgery so that you are in excellent physical condition for the actual surgery. As a bonus, you'll be ready to continue that program for the rest of your life after the surgery.

✔ Start a diet program that you stick to for several months before the surgery. This step makes it much easier to follow a diet program after the surgery. It also makes the surgery easier to perform.

✔ Drink eight 8-ounce glasses of water each day.

✔ Stop smoking permanently, starting at least eight weeks prior to surgery.

✔ Stop drinking beverages that have caffeine in them, including coffee, caffeinated tea, and soda. Check the label on any bottle you drink, and when in doubt, choose water!

✔ Attend support groups for patients undergoing bariatric surgery.

✔ Check with your surgeon about taking other medications that you are on prior to the surgery.

Knowing what to expect on the day of surgery

Your surgeon will give you detailed instructions on how to prepare and what to expect, but here are some general guidelines:

✔ The day before your surgery, you must start fasting after dinner.

✔ The surgery itself takes about two hours under general anesthesia.

✔ Most surgeries are done with the laparoscope. This permits the surgeon to view the procedure on a separate video monitor. Patients who have laparoscopic surgery have fewer complications and can return to work much quicker. They experience less infection and less pain as well.

✔ If you have gastric banding done, you will probably go home the same day.

✔ If you have gastric bypass surgery, you will spend a night at the hospital.

✔ You will receive antibiotics only if there is evidence of infection.

✔ You will need someone to drive you home after the surgery.

Charting a successful course after surgery

After the surgery is done, you continue to make the changes that allow you to lose weight and keep it off. Here are the things you have to do:

✔ Continue your diet program, preferably with the help of a dietitian. You will be eating very small amounts of food at a time, chewing thoroughly.

✔ Continue your exercise program so that as you lose weight, you lose fat and not lean tissue like muscle.

✔ Consider plastic surgery to remove the redundant skin that results from the weight loss.

✔ Go to a support group. Only people who have had the same surgery can know what you are feeling.

✔ Keep your follow-up appointments with your surgeon, dietician, and so on to continue getting the support you need.

For more information, consider picking up *Weight Loss Surgery For Dummies* by Marina S. Kurian, MD, FACS, Barbara Thompson, and Brian K. Davidson (Wiley).

Thinking about Surgery for an Obese Child or Adolescent

Obesity in children has greatly increased in the last few decades. In the United States, the percentage of children who are obese has increased from 4 percent in 1971 to 15 percent in 2007. In 2008, 4 percent of children were considered to meet the criteria for *extreme obesity* (meaning they had a body mass index of 40 or more). Obese children have a 70 percent chance of becoming obese adults.

And as obesity in children increases, so do the conditions that go along with it: high blood pressure, type 2 diabetes, high cholesterol, fatty livers, and early heart disease. Unless drastic changes are made, life expectancy in the United States will decrease as a result. Is weight loss surgery the answer? In this section, I weigh the pros and cons of surgery for kids.

Meeting some strict criteria

Just as in adults, the foundation of treatment for obesity in children is diet and exercise. But just as in adults, lifestyle changes aren't always successful. Weight loss surgery has been very effective in reducing or reversing the complications of obesity in adults, so you may assume it's the answer for kids as well. But surgery has not been proved as successful for children as for adults, and the decision to pursue surgery has to be taken very seriously.

Here are the criteria for considering weight loss surgery for children and adolescents:

- ✔ The patient has failed six months of organized attempts to improve his or her weight.
- ✔ The patient has mature bone age (meaning the bones are fully grown) so that the surgery does not affect growth.
- ✔ The patient has extreme obesity with evidence of complications of obesity like heart disease, diabetes, and high blood pressure.
- ✔ The patient will participate in psychological and medical evaluations before and after surgery.
- ✔ The patient will adhere to nutritional guidelines after surgery.
- ✔ The patient has a supportive family.

Weight loss surgery is not recommended for a young person who:

- ✔ Has a medically correctable cause of obesity
- ✔ Has a substance abuse problem
- ✔ Would not follow dietary restrictions
- ✔ Is currently pregnant or trying to become pregnant
- ✔ Does not have a supportive family

Because mature bone age is one of the criteria, weight loss surgery is not recommended in young children. Someone under the age of 16 will probably not be able to have bariatric surgery, although surgeons have operated on children as young as 12.

For adolescents, surgery would be seriously considered in the following circumstances:

✔ The patient has a body mass index (BMI) of at least 35 plus complications like high blood pressure, high cholesterol, diabetes, or heart disease. (See Chapter 6 to find out how to calculate BMI.)

✔ The patient has a BMI of 40 or more, with or without complications.

Gastric bypass is the only approved operation for adolescents in the United States. Adjustable gastric banding is done more often outside the United States.

Facing the risks

All the information I supply earlier in this chapter about the risks of gastric bypass or gastric banding apply to adolescents as well. In addition, some special considerations apply to young people:

✔ Like adults, adolescents may develop nutritional deficiencies from malabsorption after gastric bypass surgery, especially for calcium, vitamin D, folate, and B vitamins (B_1, B_6, and B_{12}). In order to continue to grow normally, these patients *must* receive vitamin supplementation. They also may develop malabsorption of fat resulting in deficiency of fat-soluble vitamins, especially A, D, E, or K. Iron malabsorption is especially important to monitor because adolescent girls are menstruating and can become anemic.

✔ Sexually active adolescents should use condoms to prevent pregnancy, especially for the first year after the surgery. A pregnancy that takes place in a patient who has not stabilized in terms of weight loss and malabsorption will be risky for both the mother and growing fetus.

Just like adults who have weight loss surgery, adolescents need to follow an exercise program and nutritional guidelines to continue to lose weight. Noncompliance is very common in adolescents.

Waiting for results

The long-term results of weight loss surgery in adolescents are just being gathered. The National Institute of Diabetes and Digestive and Kidney Diseases has created a program to try to gather this type of information. The program is called the Teen-Longitudinal Assessment of Bariatric Surgery

(Teen-LABS). It will determine the risks and benefits of weight loss surgery for adolescents.

Teen-LABS will give us a much better idea of the long-term consequences of bariatric surgery in adolescents. The program is looking at these factors:

✔ Heart risk factors and fitness

✔ Changes in hormones

✔ Sleep disorders

✔ Weight loss and body composition

✔ Kidney disease

✔ Liver function and size

✔ Risks of bariatric surgery

✔ Nutrient deficiencies

✔ Adherence to nutritional supplements

✔ Psychological and social factors.

If you want to know more information about this important program, go to the Web site of one of the medical centers in the program at www.cincinnati childrens.org/research/project/teen-labs.

Chapter 20

Putting Your Knowledge to Work: A Healthier You in Three Months

- -

- -

*I*f you have read the previous chapters in this book, you know the possible consequences if you let prediabetes turn into diabetes. I give you a lot of advice throughout the book on how to prevent that transition from happening, but what do you do day-to-day? In this chapter, I integrate the key how-to information in this book into a program that you can follow for three months. When I planned this program, I made a key assumption: that you are overweight or obese.

Before you begin this program, I suggest you establish a reward system for yourself. Every day that you follow the program exactly, give yourself a dollar. If you follow it the full 90 days, you will have $90 to spend on some non-food reward. (Decide in advance what your reward will be so your motivation is greater.)

Try to be in a very positive frame of mind when you start this program. Make sure you are ready. If you are not, you won't do well.

After you have successfully followed this three-month program, you will feel much better physically and psychologically. You may want to follow it for an additional three months, or you may be ready for some variety. Either way is fine. You can make substitutions for the foods I suggest to create a very different diet for yourself. Just make sure you keep the portions about the same so that you end up with about the same number of calories each day.

Getting Ready to Change

You need to do a few things to get ready to start this program:

✔ Let your family know what you are doing.

✔ Buy a pedometer, two 5-pound weights, and two 10-pound weights.

✔ Get rid of the foods in your house that contain the ingredients that make weight control difficult: soft drinks, foods with high fructose corn syrup, and foods with trans fats or hydrogenated oils.

✔ Stock up on the staples that I list in Chapter 15.

✔ Have some baseline studies done (see Chapter 10):

- Hemoglobin A1c

- Fasting blood glucose

- Blood pressure

- Cholesterol

- Triglycerides

- Your weight

- Your body mass index

With the exception of the hemoglobin A1c, try to do these studies every two weeks during the program. Do not weigh yourself daily because you may not see much change from day to day. (You'll definitely see change over a two-week period.) Repeat the hemoglobin A1c at the end of the three months. Record your measurements in a table so you can easily see your progress.

If you are not perfect on a particular day, don't give up in frustration. Just get back into the program the next day. A few bad days here or there are not going to affect the overall program, especially if most days are good ones.

Following the Plan

You need to learn to walk before you can run. The first month is meant to get you revved up so you can go full speed in month two. There are three elements to the change you are making: the food you are eating, the exercise you are doing, and the behavioral change you are accomplishing.

During these three months, try to eat at home as much as you can. You'll succeed much more easily if you do.

Week 1

The exercise: Wear your pedometer every day for the first week, and just let the steps add up for seven days. Divide by seven to get the number of steps per day. On Wednesday and Saturday mornings, use the 5-pound weights to perform the resistance exercises shown in Chapter 17. Repeat each exercise ten times, and then repeat each exercise ten times again.

The diet: You will eat 1,500 calories each day. The diet is very simple and easy to prepare but well-balanced so that you get all the nutrients, vitamins, and minerals you need. The emphasis is on low glycemic foods (see Chapter 16). I provide a sample menu for each week, and you can alter it to provide some variety, exchanging foods of similar nutrient and caloric quality. (I offer suggested substitutions after the sample menu.) For example, instead of ½ cup of apple juice, you can eat an apple or ¾ cups of blueberries or blackberries. Instead of 3 ounces of skinless chicken, you may eat 3 ounces of fish or 3 ounces of veal. Alternatively, so that you know you are following the program exactly, you can do the diet exactly as I have written it every day.

Here is the sample 1,500-calorie menu:

Breakfast

½ cup apple juice

1 piece whole grain toast

1 teaspoon butter

1 scrambled egg

1 cup skim milk

Lunch

3 ounces skinless chicken

½ cup cooked green beans

4 walnuts

1 slice whole grain bread

1 cup applesauce

Dinner

4 ounces lean beef

1 slice whole grain bread

1 cup cooked broccoli

½ cup peas

⅓ cantaloupe

2 tablespoons salad dressing

Salad of lettuce, tomato, onion, mushroom, celery

4 ounces low-fat yogurt

Snack

¼ cup cottage cheese

½ toasted English muffin

½ cup skim milk

Following are six substitutions that you can make for each food in this menu to give yourself a variety of tastes for the week.

Breakfast

For the apple juice:

- ✔ Apple
- ✔ ½ banana
- ✔ ¾ cup blueberries or blackberries
- ✔ 12 cherries
- ✔ ½ cup grapefruit juice
- ✔ 2 tablespoons raisins

For the whole grain toast:

- ✔ ½ cup cooked cereal
- ✔ ½ cup bran cereal
- ✔ ½ cup shredded wheat

- ½ whole wheat bagel
- 1 slice raisin bread
- 3 tablespoons Grape Nuts

For the egg:

- ¼ cup cottage cheese
- 1 ounce diet cheese
- ¼ cup egg substitute
- 3 egg whites
- 1 ounce tuna canned in water
- 1 ounce of skinless chicken or turkey

For the skim milk:

- 1 cup ½-percent milk
- 1 cup 1 percent milk
- 1 cup nonfat or low-fat buttermilk
- ¾ cup plain non-fat yogurt
- ½ cup evaporated skim milk
- ⅓ cup dry non-fat milk

Lunch

For the skinless chicken:

- 3 ounces lean pork
- 3 ounces lean veal (except no veal cutlet)
- 3 ounces wild game, such as venison, rabbit, or squirrel
- 3 ounces pheasant, duck, or goose
- 3 ounces fresh fish
- 3 ounces tuna canned in water

For the cooked green beans:

- ½ medium artichoke
- ½ cup cooked or 1 cup raw carrots

✔ ½ cup cooked cauliflower

✔ ½ cup cooked eggplant

✔ ½ cup cooked pea pods

✔ ½ cup cooked summer squash

For the walnuts:

✔ ¼ avocado

✔ 12 almonds

✔ 2 tablespoons cashews

✔ 4 pecans

✔ 20 peanuts

✔ 2 tablespoons sunflower seeds

The dinner and snack foods can be substituted in the same way: a fruit for a fruit; a vegetable for a vegetable; a meat, fish, or poultry for a meat, fish, or poultry; dairy for dairy; a starch (like bread) for a starch (like cereal).

The behavioral change: Do nothing while you are eating besides eating: no television, no Web surfing, no talking on the phone, and no reading.

Week 2

The exercise: Do the same exercise as the first week but add 500 steps each day to the average daily steps of the first week. If you averaged 3,500 daily steps in week 1, for example, do 4,000 daily. On Wednesday and Saturday mornings, use the 5-pound weights to perform the resistance exercises shown in Chapter 17. Do the resistance exercises for 12 repetitions instead of 10.

The diet: Follow the same program as week 1.

The behavioral change: Keep a daily journal listing the food you eat, the exercise you do, and your mood. See Chapter 16 for ideas about how to keep a food record.

At the end of week 2, repeat the baseline measurements I describe in the "Getting Ready to Change" section earlier in the chapter (except the hemoglobin A1c).

Week 3

The exercise: Add 1,000 steps to the daily average of week 1. On Wednesday and Saturday mornings, use the 5-pound weights to perform the resistance exercises shown in Chapter 17. Do the resistance exercises for 15 repetitions instead of 12.

The diet: Follow the same program as week 1.

The behavioral change: Add water to your diet. Drink water before, during, and after each meal.

Week 4

The exercise: Add 1,500 steps to the daily average of week 1. On Wednesday and Saturday mornings, use the 5-pound weights to perform the resistance exercises shown in Chapter 17. Add a third set of the resistance exercises so you're doing 15 repetitions of each exercise three times.

The diet: Follow the same program as week 1.

The behavioral change: Slow down your eating to make the food last. Put down your fork or spoon between each bite, and don't pick it up until you have swallowed the food. Chew each bite for a long time.

At the end of week 4, repeat the baseline measurements I describe in the "Getting Ready to Change" section earlier in the chapter (except the hemoglobin A1c).

Week 5

The exercise: Add 2,000 steps to the daily average of week 1. On Wednesday and Saturday mornings, use the 5-pound weights to perform the resistance exercises shown in Chapter 17. Do the resistance exercises the same number of times as in week 4.

The diet: Follow the same program as week 1.

The behavioral change: Find a single place to eat all your food: the designated eating place. It should be a place where you do nothing but eat, such as the dinner table or the kitchen table.

Week 6

The exercise: Add 2,500 steps to the daily average of week 1. On Wednesday and Saturday mornings, perform the resistance exercises shown in Chapter 17. For the resistance exercises, start using the 10-pound weights but do only two sets of ten repetitions.

The diet: Follow the same program as week 1.

The behavioral change: Eat according to a schedule to avoid unplanned eating. Eat three meals a day and a snack daily, or take a little from a meal to have a second snack.

At the end of week 6, repeat the baseline measurements I describe in the "Getting Ready to Change" section earlier in the chapter (except the hemoglobin A1c).

Week 7

The exercise: Add 3,000 steps to the daily average of week 1. On Wednesday and Saturday mornings, perform the resistance exercises shown in Chapter 17. Using the 10-pound weights, do two sets of 12 repetitions.

The diet: Follow the same program as week 1.

The behavioral change: Use smaller plates and bowls so that your portions, which are undoubtedly less than you are used to, will appear sufficient.

Week 8

The exercise: Add 3,500 steps to the daily average of week 1. On Wednesday and Saturday mornings, perform the resistance exercises shown in Chapter 17. Using the 10-pound weights, do two sets of 15 repetitions.

The diet: Follow the same program as week 1.

The behavioral change: Keep all food that you are not eating in the kitchen. Don't leave plates of food on counters. Keep leftovers in opaque containers.

At the end of week 8, repeat the baseline measurements I describe in the "Getting Ready to Change" section earlier in the chapter (except the hemoglobin A1c).

Week 9

The exercise: Add 4,000 steps to the daily average of week 1. On Wednesday and Saturday mornings, perform the resistance exercises shown in Chapter 17. Using the 10-pound weights, do three sets of ten repetitions.

The diet: Follow the same program as week 1.

The behavioral change: Don't dispense food to others, and don't serve meals family style.

Week 10

The exercise: Add 4,500 steps to the daily average of week 1. On Wednesday and Saturday mornings, perform the resistance exercises shown in Chapter 17. Using the 10-pound weights, do three sets of 12 repetitions.

The diet: Follow the same program as week 1.

The behavioral change: At the market, buy from a list, carry only enough money for the food on that list, and avoid aisles containing loose foods other than fruits and vegetables.

At the end of week 10, repeat the baseline measurements I describe in the "Getting Ready to Change" section earlier in the chapter (except the hemoglobin A1c).

Week 11

The exercise: Add 5,000 steps to the daily average of week 1. By this point you should be at or very close to 10,000 steps a day. That is the goal. If you are there, you can stay at that level or do more if you want to, but not less.

On Wednesday and Saturday mornings, perform the resistance exercises shown in Chapter 17. Using the 10-pound weights, do three sets of 15 repetitions. You are also at your resistance goal. You can do more repetitions or more sets if you desire, but if you are doing this much, you are accomplishing what you need to.

The diet: Follow the same program as week 1.

The behavioral change: Do not clean your plate. If you can learn to leave food, you may learn to stop eating when you are full.

Week 12

The exercise: You are at or near your goal. Stay at the week 11 level of aerobic and resistance exercises, or do more if you have the need.

The diet: Follow the same program as week 1.

The behavioral change: Avoid fast food as much as possible. If you eat out, keep salad dressing on the side, limit alcohol to one drink, and avoid bread.

At the end of week 12, repeat the baseline measurements I describe in the "Getting Ready to Change" section earlier in the chapter, including the hemoglobin A1c.

Applauding Your Accomplishments

If you follow this plan closely, you will accomplish many of the following goals by the end of three months:

- You will lose between 10 and 15 pounds.
- You will reduce your waistline by1 to 2 inches, most of which is the visceral fat that leads to coronary artery disease.
- You will significantly increase your stamina so that you can perform at a high level for much longer.
- You will significantly increase your strength so that you can easily hoist that carry-on bag into the overhead bin.
- You will greatly improve the quality of your life so that you feel much better about yourself.
- Your fasting blood glucose will fall by 15 to 25 mg/dl, and your blood glucose after eating will fall by 40 to 60 mg/dl.
- Your total cholesterol will fall by 20 to 40 mg/dl, and your good cholesterol will rise by 10 to 20 mg/dl.
- Your hemoglobin A1c will fall at least 1 percent.
- Your body mass index (BMI) may fall from the obese range into the overweight range.
- Your blood pressure will fall by 15 to 20 mg systolic and by 5 to 10 mg diastolic.

✔ You will feel much more self-assured and able to do whatever you set your mind to.

✔ You will feel much sexier, and other people will think so too!

✔ Your thinking will be much clearer.

✔ You will be sleeping much better and feeling much less tired during the day.

✔ If you had sleep apnea, you will be sleeping soundly.

✔ Your joints will not hurt nearly as much.

✔ You will be playing the violin beautifully. (Just kidding.)

Knowledge about prediabetes and diabetes is expanding so fast that great advances are arriving almost daily. Some of these advances may be just what you need. If you can put off developing diabetes for some years, you put off developing the complications as well. You benefit from the *legacy effect,* where control of your blood glucose for several years slows down the development of complications for years after that, even if you later lose your control.

Part VI
The Part of Tens

The 5th Wave

By Rich Tennant

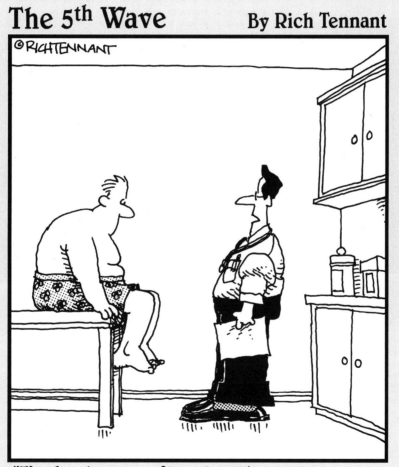

"I'm having you fitted with a monitoring device that will help reduce blood glucose during meals by automatically signaling the brain to reduce food absorption. It's called a belt."

In this part . . .

This part is an opportunity to give you some key tools for eliminating prediabetes. First, I expose and rebut some common myths about prediabetes. Next, I offer more than ten staples to keep in your kitchen so that you are always ready to cook and eat the right thing. Finally, I offer advice for helping your child overcome prediabetes and live a long and healthy life.

Chapter 21

Ten Myths about Prediabetes

*L*ike all conditions that affect more than 50 million people, prediabetes is bound to be associated with a lot of myths. Think of it like that old childhood game of telephone, where one person whispers something into the ear of the next person and it goes around the circle until the last person says what he heard. Even without trying to change what is said, the last person rarely says anything like what the first person said.

Now add to the mix the natural inclination in this capitalist society to make money. People come up with a lot of misinformation in an effort to convince you to turn over your hard-earned dollars to them. By reading this chapter, you will save yourself way more than the price of this book, proving again how smart you were to buy it. (You did buy it, didn't you?)

In this chapter, I address just a few of the many myths surrounding prediabetes. If you have a myth that you think I should include in this book, e-mail it to me at drrubin@drrubin.com. I just may use it in a future edition.

I Have Borderline Diabetes

There is no such thing as *borderline* diabetes. For that matter, you do not just have "a little sugar." As I explain in Chapter 1, diabetes, prediabetes, and the normal state are all well-defined by lab results:

> ✔ **Normal:** A normal fasting blood glucose test result is less than 100 mg/dl, and a normal blood glucose level two hours after eating glucose is less than 140 mg/dl.

✔ **Prediabetes:** A fasting blood glucose test result between 100 and 125 mg/dl defines prediabetes, as does a glucose level between 140 to 199 mg/dl two hours after eating glucose. (These test results must occur on more than one occasion to secure a diagnosis.)

✔ **Diabetes:** Diabetes is defined as a fasting blood glucose of 126 mg/dl or more or a blood glucose of 200 mg/dl or more two hours after eating glucose. (Again, these results must occur on more than one occasion.)

Here's where things get a little confusing: Some people with prediabetes can develop complications of diabetes. But this fact just shows that the definitions need work. Until they are altered, you can avoid a lot of confusion by using them exactly as they are stated here.

My Biggest Problem Is Elevated Blood Sugars

Prediabetes is defined by the elevated blood glucose. It would be great if that was the only problem occurring in your body. But an abnormal blood glucose is often secondary to obesity, and a lot more is probably happening that you can't see. For example:

✔ Your blood pressure may be elevated.

✔ Your blood cholesterol may be high with lots of bad (LDL) cholesterol and not enough good (HDL) cholesterol.

✔ Coronary artery disease is gradually occurring.

✔ You may be starting to damage your eyes and kidneys.

✔ You may be developing arthritis in your joints because of all the weight that you are carrying on them.

You need to look at all these problems — not just the blood glucose. In Chapter 10, I talk about all the areas you should be considering. Get a good eye exam. Have your doctor test your kidney function, your blood pressure, and your *lipids* (total cholesterol, good cholesterol, bad cholesterol, and triglycerides). Think of your body as a car. To keep it in good shape, you wouldn't just check the brakes and forget about the engine, the tires, the lights, and so forth.

I Can't Eat Anything Fun

If you've read Chapter 16, I hope you've changed you mind about this one. If you haven't read it yet, I highly recommend it. The recipes in that chapter are as good as anything from any fine restaurant, and they are all good for you.

Some food items, like luncheon meats and foods full of trans fats, simply should not be on your plate — they'll take years off your life. You also don't want to eat foods that your grandmother would not recognize as food. (This includes any item with 25 ingredients, many of which are coloring agents or preservatives.)

You want to emphasize low glycemic foods that contain fiber and are, therefore, not highly processed. (I explain what low glycemic foods are in Chapter 16.) You want to eat a variety of delicious fresh fruits and vegetables.

You can even eat some dessert. (See . . . I'm not such a killjoy!) Just keep your total calories each day at or below the calories you burn up daily so that you don't gain weight.

Eating a healthy diet does not need to be a drudgery. Enjoy your food, and make sure you have good company when you eat.

I Have to Get Thin to Be Healthy

If you are currently overweight or obese, it's unlikely that you will ever become thin. All I ask of you is that you lose enough weight so that you don't have to worry about developing diabetes if you are prediabetic. If you already have type 2 diabetes, you may need to lose a little more. I want you to reach a *healthy* weight at which your blood glucose levels are normal. That healthy weight is often a lot heavier than your so-called "ideal weight" (see Chapter 6).

As I explain in Chapter 6, your *body mass index* (BMI) is key to determining whether you are overweight. You are considered to be thin if your body mass index is below 18. From 18 to 24.9 is normal, from 25 to 29.9 is overweight, and 30 or above is obese.

If you wish to look like a fashion model, that's entirely up to you, but looking like a fashion model isn't so great either. Models often get that thin by starving themselves, smoking, and eating a terribly unbalanced diet.

Some studies seem to indicate that people who are underweight live longer than people who are normal in weight. But to quote from *Porgy and Bess,* "Who calls dat livin?"

It is possible to be overweight and still be healthy if you exercise regularly. Some studies have shown that a mildly overweight person can actually live longer than a thin person.

The old cliché goes, "You can never be too thin or too rich." From my perspective, it's only half right. I leave it to you to guess which half.

Exercise Is Dangerous for Me

On the contrary. As Chapter 17 conclusively proves, exercise can turn pre-diabetes into normal metabolism. Assuming that you are reasonably healthy (and that if you are starting an exercise program over age 40 you have checked with your doctor), there is no limitation to the amount of exercise you can do. I am not suggesting you start by climbing Mt. Everest. In Chapter 20, I provide a very reasonable schedule for building yourself up so that you can eventually climb Mt. Everest, but you need to start with a flat walk.

You will be amazed and very proud of what you are capable of doing. Today you may think that a mile is an incredible distance. After a few months of training, a mile will seem like no big deal.

You ultimately want to do very vigorous exercise, if that's possible for you, because that's how you make the greatest gains. And if you are really short on time, a few minutes of vigorous exercise accomplishes what 30 minutes or an hour of less vigorous exercise can do.

Don't stop with aerobic exercise. Resistance training is equally important to build up your muscles and your stamina. It will allow you to easily put your carry-on luggage in the overhead rack and even help others to lift theirs.

You need to make exercise as much a part of your life as eating your meals and going to the bathroom. Exercise gives you a legal high that you shouldn't miss.

Vitamins and Other Supplements Can Help Me

I spend much of Chapter 18 destroying this myth. The number of so-called *health enhancers* is becoming enormous. One of the unfortunate effects of the

Internet is to provide a huge space on which the purveyors of quackery can try to convince you to buy their products. Based on the story of one person who took the product and changed from an overweight couch potato to a lean, mean health machine, these people ask you to send in your money.

One of my new patients was taking more than 25 supplements and vitamins and still felt lousy. I showed him that scientific studies had failed to prove that any of the pills had value. In fact, studies showed how supplements could be hurting him. He agreed to stop taking them and saw an immediate improvement in his health (and his bank account).

Not all supplements are worthless, of course. But if they truly have value, they must pass the test of a *double-blind study* where everyone gets a pill that looks the same but half contain the supplement and half a placebo. Neither the patients nor the doctors know which is which until all the data is collected about how the patients responded. Each supplement is touted as having a special healing property. If it does, the people who actually received the supplement should do significantly better with respect to that property than the people who received a placebo.

The trouble is that the U.S. Food and Drug Administration (FDA) has no control over these supplements. They are not considered drugs, which the FDA does control. And the FDA is overwhelmed with the work it is already doing. It hardly has time to police the claims of these supplements and vitamins, which come out at the rate of several a week.

Bottom line: Don't just start taking supplements. Discuss them with your doctor or try to find published studies that use the double-blind technique I describe in this section to demonstrate the product's value.

I Have to Buy Special Machines to Monitor My Status

Most of these machines have the same value as the supplements I describe in the preceding section. (In other words, not much.) You really need only two machines to evaluate your medical status: a glucose meter and a blood pressure cuff.

If you have prediabetes, you want to occasionally check your blood glucose to make sure that it is staying below the definition of diabetes. Equally important, you should be measuring your blood pressure to make sure it is normal, especially if you take blood pressure medication.

You may have heard of the *continuous glucose monitor,* which you wear on your body. It checks your blood glucose every 5 minutes and alerts you if your glucose is above or below levels that you set. If you have prediabetes, it's unlikely that you will ever go above or below those levels. You don't need that much information.

I Need to Take Diet Pills

In Chapter 18, which is all about medications for prediabetes, I say absolutely nothing about diet pills. The reason is that for the most part, they are worthless. Only a few drugs are authorized by the FDA for weight loss, and they have little value. Here are some of the problems with the available weight loss drugs:

- ✔ They often raise your blood pressure and heart rate.

- ✔ They may cause *tolerance* (the continued need for bigger doses) and dependence to develop.

- ✔ Weight loss is minimal compared with a placebo.

- ✔ They are approved for just a few weeks' use but are often taken for months or years with little effect.

- ✔ They can cause you to become agitated.

- ✔ No weight loss drug has ever been shown to prevent a disease state — only to cause some minimal weight loss.

- ✔ Some diet drugs cause significant side effects like gas, fatty stools, and frequent bowel movements.

- ✔ Some diet drugs cause precancerous changes, pancreatitis, and other abnormalities.

Over 30 years of medical practice, I have had patients ask me for every diet pill that has ever been produced. I used to give them the pills, hoping that each one would work long-term. I have never seen pills work for very long. Sooner or later the patient stops taking them, eats too much for them to work, or does so well with diet and exercise that the pills are unnecessary. I no longer prescribe diet pills to anyone.

Save your money and your health. Don't bother with diet pills.

A Week at a Health Spa Is All I Need

Miracles do not occur at health spas. You can't take an individual who is significantly overweight and turn him into a slim and trim person. The person took years to get into that state, and he needs at least months (maybe even a year or more) to reverse the situation.

I am not against going to a spa, but you have to understand its limitations. You usually get food that you would never cook for yourself. You do hours and hours of physical activity that you would never have time for at home.

A spa is a vacation from real life. It tends to be very expensive, which is somewhat ironic considering the minimal portions of food that are often served. Instead of sitting on a couch relaxing, you go from one exercise class to another. You often come home exhausted from a spa.

You may get massages, which are nice but hardly solve your problem. You get treatments with such things as cucumbers on your face that are of questionable value. You may lose a few pounds, but you usually quickly regain them when you return home.

Enjoy your week at the spa, but don't count on reversing your prediabetes there.

I'm On My Own

The fact is that lots of people want to help you, starting with your family. They need to be engaged in making the right kinds of foods and helping you to make the right choices. Often, if one member of a family is obese and has prediabetes, several other family members have the same problem. Try to work together with them to follow good eating habits and do regular exercise. The behavioral changes that I suggest in Chapter 16 are even more powerful if all family members do them together.

Next is your doctor. He can make sure you are in good health before you start an exercise program. He can test you for the important measurements like blood pressure, kidney function, and cholesterol levels and interpret them for you. If you smoke, he can help you to stop.

Then there is the dietitian, who can offer a sensible plan for weight loss. She can work with you so that you continue to eat the things you enjoy but not the amounts that are causing your weight gain.

Another source of help is a psychologist, who can help you to understand some of the issues that motivate you to do unhealthful things.

Then there are support groups. It can be very helpful to hear how others have coped with the things you are going through. And your experience can help others. You feel less alone. You can vent and know that someone is listening. If money is an issue, keep in mind that support groups are often free. The only problem with support groups is that often there is no expert to guide the group, so not all the information you hear may be accurate. You can find support groups for just about any issue that you have. Here are some ways to find one:

- Ask your doctor or therapist.
- Contact a mental health organization.
- Check the phonebook under *mental health* or *counseling*.
- Contact local community centers or libraries.
- Get recommendations from friends or relatives.
- Search the Internet.

Numerous resources are available to you, and numerous people are just waiting to offer their expertise to help you. Don't waste another minute!

Chapter 22

(More Than) Ten Staples to Keep in Your Kitchen

In This Chapter
▶ Enjoying vegetables
▶ Staying strong with protein
▶ Finishing with fruit
▶ Garnishing with herbs and spices

*1*t's a lot easier to eat the foods that are good for you if they are easily available to you. And it's a lot easier to avoid the foods that are bad for you if they are out of sight and out of the house. Plenty of delicious foods will keep well in your fridge and pantry. Why not have them right there where you can prepare a delicious meal without a lot of hassle?

If you need recipes to use these staples, try my book *Diabetes Cookbook For Dummies,* 2nd Edition (Wiley). The recipes in that book are not just for people with diabetes but for anyone who wants to eat delicious, healthy food.

Make sure you buy things when they are in season. If you buy out of season, the food is coming from a long distance and you are paying for transportation. You are definitely not paying for taste because these traveling vegetables are grown to survive shipment and to last a long time.

Green Vegetables

Salad is more than just lettuce and tomatoes. Creative chefs have turned salads into a main course. If you do start with lettuce, choose a dark variety because it contains more nutrients. Here are a variety of greens for your kitchen that will provide a variety of nutrients:

- Arugula, also known as *rocket* or *roquette*
- Boston lettuce, also called *butterhead*
- Chicory, which includes *radicchio, escarole,* and *frisée*
- Endive
- Watercress

Store salad greens in the vegetable bin of the refrigerator. Compact lettuce is best stored intact, but loose leaf has to be washed, drained, and stored in a plastic bag to keep it fresh.

Tomatoes

Tomatoes are one of the most delicious vegetables you can eat. There are so many varieties that they could easily fill a book, but I prefer the heirloom varieties to the more modern tomato hybrids. Don't buy tomatoes in the winter, when they come from thousands of miles away, are exceedingly expensive, and are not grown for taste. (Instead, they're grown for the ability to withstand a long trip.)

In most areas, tomatoes are in season from July to September. They come in all colors representing all kinds of nutrients, but the main ones are vitamins C, A, and K. You can also get some of your daily potassium needs, as well as some fiber. And the best thing is that despite how good they taste, tomatoes are low in calories.

The best tomato is one you pick from the tomato plant that you have grown. In warm climates, a few tomato plants can keep an entire family eating tomatoes all summer.

Tomatoes keep beautifully in the refrigerator. They are filled with *antioxidants,* which protect against cancer. Organic tomatoes seem to have more antioxidants than non-organic ones. Eating lots of tomatoes has also been found to lower cholesterol levels.

If you buy canned tomatoes, look for a variety made in the United States. Doing so can help you avoid getting a lot of lead along with your tomatoes.

Proteins

You can get your protein from a variety of sources, which I cover in this section.

Fresh meat, fish, and poultry

Unless they are frozen, meat, fish, and poultry do not keep very well. You should buy these items the day you plan to eat them. They are, of course, the most expensive way to get your protein. To keep the fat low, remove the skin. When you cook them, don't use breading. Also, be sure to keep your intake of goose and duck to a minimum because they are so fatty.

If you're going to eat beef, get the lean variety, with less than 15 percent fat. Also, buy "choice" or "select" grades of beef rather than "prime" because prime has the most fat. Purchase lean ham, lean pork, and lean veal, but remember that even lean ham has a lot of sodium.

Meats that are especially lean (and unusual) include emu, buffalo, and ostrich. They are low in fat and saturated fat. Wild game is also better than farm animals because it is much less fatty.

Canned fish

Fresh fish is a great way to get your protein, but let's face it: You can't go to the grocery store every day, and fish just doesn't last long in your refrigerator.

Canned fish is an excellent way to have fish available at any time. The best are canned salmon and canned tuna fish. Make sure you check the food label for the amount of sodium and for packaging in water. Oil-packed canned fish is very high in calories. The other thing you want to check the label for is the number of servings per can. Just because the can is small does not mean it is one serving. More often it contains two servings, so you have to share or save the other half for another day.

Canned fish offers the same health benefits as fresh fish. The oily fishes are protective against heart disease. Canned albacore tuna has the most omega-3 fatty acid, the substance that is protective. When you drain the water, the oil remains in the fish because the oil and the water don't mix. Tuna packed in oil is a different story, however. The oils in the tuna mix with the added oil, and if it is drained, some of the omega-3s are lost.

Canned salmon also provides plenty of omega-3s. Look for boneless, skinless varieties and the more tasty King salmon. Make sure the salmon is wild, not farmed. This way you can have wild salmon all year, not just during the salmon season.

Dairy products

Dairy products, including milk, cheese, and yogurt, keep longer than fresh meat, fish, or poultry and are a good source of protein. Just be sure to stick to low fat varieties.

If you can't drink cow's milk because of the lactose, soy milk is a very good substitute. An added bonus: It keeps a lot longer than cow's milk.

Eggs

Eggs had a bad reputation for a long time. Ever since people started checking their cholesterol, they have avoided eggs because each egg contains about 300 mg of cholesterol. But eggs are also a great source of protein, and they keep very well in the refrigerator.

An egg has only about 75 kilocalories and is packed with nutrients. In addition to the protein, you get choline, folate, iron, and zinc. You can reduce the cholesterol easily by getting rid of one yolk and eating two whites for each yolk.

There are countless ways you can use eggs in your diet, from the morning omelet to a seafood soufflé. Just stay away from the additions that make eggs so high in calories, like Hollandaise sauce.

If you have concerns about egg safety, rest assured that properly cooking eggs makes them very safe. Bacteria are killed as the egg cooks. Make sure no liquid egg is left when your eggs are cooked, and you will have destroyed any bacteria that were hanging around.

Beans

"Beans, beans, the musical fruit — the more you eat, the more you toot!"

I learned that rule when I was about 5 years old and confirmed it the first time I had beans to eat. Beyond that, beans are a great food.

Beans are an excellent way to get your protein. They are low in fat and high in protein. They contain a lot of fiber, which lowers cholesterol and slows the uptake of carbohydrates. Dried beans are available all year and are inexpensive. They have to be soaked for six to eight hours, so you have to plan ahead. They taste bland by themselves but take on the taste of whatever food they are mixed with, such as tomatoes.

Canned beans, which are precooked, are immediately available for a speedy, delicious meal. But watch out for the extra sodium in canned beans. Read the label!

Nuts and seeds

The fats in nuts are mostly the good kind: monounsaturated and polyunsaturated fats, which help your heart. The best nuts include almonds, cashews, pistachios, walnuts, and peanuts. Nuts also contain a lot of vitamin E and fiber. And, of course, nuts keep for a long time.

The U.S. Food and Drug Administration (FDA) has approved a health claim for nuts that states, "Scientific evidence suggests but does not prove that eating 1.5 oz per day of most nuts as a part of a diet low in saturated fats and cholesterol may reduce the risk of heart disease and cholesterol." The claim is approved for almonds, hazelnuts, pecans, peanuts, some pine nuts, pistachios, and walnuts because these nuts contain less than 4 grams of saturated fat per 50 grams. Flax seeds, pumpkin seeds, and sunflower seeds also offer these benefits.

While nuts and seeds are a great source of vitamin E, the oil in them starts to turn rancid after they are removed from their shells. If you buy nuts and seeds in their shells, they can last up to a year.

Seeds and nuts are calorie dense, so you have to be moderate in your intake of these foods. You should eat no more than 1 to 2 ounces daily, and make sure they are unsalted.

Berries, Apples, and Other Non-starchy Fruits

One of my favorite times of year is the berry season. It begins about June and continues until the fall. During that time you have a choice of raspberries, strawberries, loganberries, currants, gooseberries, cranberries, lingonberries, and my granddaughter's favorite: blueberries.

A cup of berries packs a lot nutrition and fiber for very few kilocalories (less than 100). You get substances called *phytochemicals* and *flavonoids* that fight cancer. You get other substances that help your vision. The substance that gives blueberries their color, called *anthocyanin,* has been shown to prolong the mental capacity of laboratory animals and may do the same in humans.

You are much better off getting your berries at the source or at a farmer's market than in the supermarket. In terms of taste, the closer you are to where the berries are grown, the better. If you can find a place where you can pick your own, that's ideal. (My granddaughter tastes every other berry, so picking our own becomes especially economical.)

Out of season, frozen berries are an excellent choice. They also last a lot longer than fresh berries.

Don't forget apples, pears, plums, peaches, apricots, grapes, and other non-starchy fruits. They are full of fiber, have few kilocalories, and make wonderful desserts. The banana is a starchy fruit, so limit yourself to half a banana at a time.

Olive Oil

Many studies tout the benefits of eating the *Mediterranean diet* — the type of diet followed by people living around the Mediterranean Sea (the Spanish, French, Italians, and Greeks). Some scientists believe that the entire benefit of this diet hinges on the use of olive oil.

Olive oil is high in monounsaturated fatty acids as well as antioxidants. *Extra virgin olive oil,* the olive oil from the first pressing of the olives, is especially high in these healthy compounds. It's the least processed oil and is *cold pressed,* meaning it's obtained without using heat.

Olive oil keeps best in a cool, dark place. When it is exposed to oxygen, it becomes rancid. Some people suggest decanting a small amount of olive oil for immediate use and putting the rest away. Others suggest filling the space above the oil with a spray that is also used to preserve wine.

Olive oil may have the following health benefits (not all of which have been proved):

- Lowering blood pressure
- Preventing or inhibiting cancer
- Preventing coronary artery disease

- ✔ Lessening the severity of asthma and arthritis
- ✔ Benefiting people with breast, prostate, and endometrial cancer

Herbs and Spices

There is no better way to add taste to your food (without adding a lot of salt) than to add herbs and spices. Fresh is best, but fresh herbs and spices don't keep long so having a bunch of dried herbs and spices on hand makes great sense. Try them on different foods and see how you change the taste. Here are some I recommend stocking:

- ✔ Allspice
- ✔ Basil
- ✔ Cayenne pepper
- ✔ Chili powder
- ✔ Cilantro
- ✔ Cinnamon
- ✔ Cloves
- ✔ Cumin
- ✔ Dill
- ✔ Garlic powder
- ✔ Garlic salt
- ✔ Ginger
- ✔ Nutmeg
- ✔ Onion powder
- ✔ Oregano
- ✔ Paprika
- ✔ Parsley
- ✔ Red pepper flakes
- ✔ Rosemary
- ✔ Sage

Chapter 23

Ten Things to Teach Your Prediabetic Child

Children start learning shortly after they are born. You want to teach your child good exercise habits, good eating habits, and good resting habits from the youngest age. Your child will likely try to emulate you in everything she does, so if you model good habits, chances are she'll follow them.

Try to include your child in all the decisions you make related to her health. Ask questions like: Shall we hike or go biking today? Should we buy the green beans, the broccoli, or the asparagus? Should we have the salmon, the tuna, or some chili for supper? Give your child two or more healthy choices. That way, no matter what she decides, she will benefit.

Also try to do healthy things together. One of my patients, who did little exercise, complained that both her sons were heavy. They were embarrassed and introverted. I suggested that she start an exercise program and invite them to join her. Both sons soon lost their excess fat, and both joined their track team, where they became leaders. My patient and her husband, who also joined in the exercise, lost a significant amount of weight as well and felt much better physically and mentally.

Diabetes Need Not Be Devastating

If your child is prediabetic, you never want him to become diabetic, so this lesson may seem a strange way to start this chapter. But your child may be terrified of what life as a diabetic would be like, and your goal here is to ease his stress.

Your child simply needs to know that if he does become diabetic, the disease is controllable. Using diet, exercise, and perhaps medication, people with diabetes can live normal lives.

People with diabetes can excel in every field, from sports to politics to the art world to private business. As I write these words, a new Supreme Court justice — Sonia Sotomayor — is headline news, and she has managed her diabetes all her life.

The key thing to teach your child is that he can thrive even with diabetes. In fact, some people with diabetes are healthier than people who don't have the diagnosis because the people with diabetes follow a much healthier program of diet and exercise.

Diabetes Is Not Inevitable

As important as the first lesson in this chapter is, the second lesson is even more so. Your child should understand that type 2 diabetes is, in many cases, a choice. This isn't *always* true, of course — plenty of people with type 2 diabetes are slim and exercise a great deal. But for the most part, type 2 diabetes is a lifestyle disease. You can choose to exercise for an hour every day and eat small portions of highly nourishing foods, or not.

Your child needs to be as far away from diabetes as possible. That means eliminating prediabetes. You may have to set some fairly rigid rules to achieve that goal. If your child pushes back, just remember that setting rules indicates that you care.

Here are some basic rules to rapidly move your child away from prediabetes:

- A maximum of two hours of looking at screens daily
- No fast food restaurants until prediabetes is gone
- A minimum of one hour of exercise daily
- More fruits and vegetables and less meat and fat

These few simple steps should put your child well on his way to normal, healthy metabolism and freedom from illness.

Now Is the Time to Act

Your child should understand that the earlier prediabetes is dealt with, the more easily it can be reversed. Here are a few reasons for acting now:

- ✔ After bad habits about food, exercise, and rest are ingrained, those habits are very tough to break.

- ✔ Good exercise habits are developed much more easily at a young age. Exercise is fun, and children love to have fun.

- ✔ It's a lot easier to lose the small amount of excess weight that a small child carries than the much larger amount of excess weight a preteen or teenager may carry. In fact, some small children outgrow the weight and don't have a problem after they get taller.

- ✔ Children generally want to fit in, and overweight kids have a tougher time doing so. When it comes to sports, social events, and even friendships, weight matters. Even as a young adult, excess weight can play a role in whether you get into the college of your choice or land the job you really want.

- ✔ By acting early to overcome prediabetes, your child has plenty of time to gain self-confidence. He develops a positive attitude that spills over into many areas of his life.

Don't waste another minute! Get started immediately!

You Can Comfort and Reward Yourself without Food

The comfort value of food is taught to children at a very young age. When they fall and start to cry, they are offered a cookie. When they do something especially noteworthy, they are rewarded with an ice cream cone. When they do something bad or don't eat their vegetables, their dessert is withheld. The powerful message this sends is that sweet, high carbohydrate food is the biggest reward and is associated with positive feelings connecting the parent and the child.

This connection between good actions and high carb food rewards should never be established. Early on, you should decide on other non-food rewards like spending extra time with your child, putting a quarter into a piggy bank, or buying a present appropriate to the value of the deed. Rewards are important motivators, but food rewards are counterproductive.

If your child earns a significant amount of money from doing the right thing, let him use it any way he wants so that he feels the effort was worth his trouble. If you choose how to spend it, he may not feel the reward was his.

Healthy Food Can Taste Great

As soon as my granddaughter started eating solid foods, my daughter fed her good fruits and vegetables that she prepared herself. She also fed her small amounts of chicken and fish. As a result, my granddaughter loves fruits, vegetables, poultry, and fish. She has no particular interest in sweets. She has learned that the taste of fresh food is far superior to highly processed baked sweets.

Any child can learn this lesson, especially at a young age. It takes more effort on the part of the parent because it's easier to heat a jar of baby food than to bake a sweet potato or some fish. But the payoff is worth the effort.

I offer many suggestions in this book for ways to turn around poor eating habits. When you have kids, one of the best things you can do is grow some of your own vegetables or take your child to a farm where you can pick them. Encourage your child to taste the vegetables immediately after you pick them, at the height of their flavor. You may not believe that a carrot can be sweeter than an ice cream cone, but you would be surprised.

Vegetables Are Delicious

From artichokes to zucchini, vegetables are nutritious, delicious foods. Children need to know that, and you need to teach them because TV shows and commercials certainly don't. The best thing you can do is eat vegetables every day yourself, and make a point to show your child how much you enjoy them.

The way vegetables are prepared often determines if a child will eat them. I'm not saying that you should bread and deep-fry every vegetable so it resembles a fast-food product! Consider these possibilities:

- Kids often enjoy vegetables that are stir-fried with a little peanut oil or another oil.
- Vegetables can be pureed into great-tasting soups.

✔ Pureed vegetables can also be added to pasta sauce.

✔ Most children will happily drink vegetable juice.

✔ If my granddaughter is any indication, acorn squash can become a kid favorite. (She especially loves it with peas.)

Potatoes are one vegetable that I recommend avoiding because they have a very high glycemic index (see Chapter 16). They are absorbed rapidly and raise your blood glucose rapidly. Also, they are often served fried or with butter and sour cream. So don't push the potatoes.

Water Is Vital

Children need to learn how vital water is to their health. Avoid starting your child on soft drinks at all costs. Encourage her to drink water before, during, and after each meal. Feel free to make disparaging remarks about the worthlessness of soft drinks, flavored drinks, and even dietetic drinks.

Children should appreciate that the best thirst quencher is water. Make sure your child has easy access to water all day long. For very young kids, that may mean placing a stool near the sink or keeping a pitcher of water on the lowest shelf of the refrigerator so they can help themselves.

Explain to your child that dehydration will prevent her from performing at her best both mentally and physically. She needs to know that it's most important to drink after sweating. If she goes from gym class to an academic subject and is not hydrated, she likely won't perform well in class or on tests.

The fact that your child is growing makes it even more important that she be well hydrated. Dehydration can occur much more rapidly in children than in adults. They are less aware of thirst than adults, so they can become dehydrated more easily.

Get your child in the habit of drinking water all the time. Doing so establishes a habit that yields benefits through her whole life.

People Are Supposed to Move

Children should be aware of the philosophy "a sound mind in a sound body." You need to inspire your child to actively work on both, and exercise is a great way to do so.

Just like adults, children derive numerous benefits from exercise. Here's a short list you can share with your child:

- Exercise builds and maintains healthy bones, muscles, and joints.
- Exercise helps you feel better about yourself.
- Exercise reduces feelings of stress.
- Exercise can help you feel more ready to learn in school.
- Exercise helps you maintain a healthy weight.
- Exercise helps you sleep better at night.

Most importantly, know that your child will exercise if you do. So get out there and set an example!

We All Need Rest

As important as exercise is, rest is equally important. Rest allows your body to rejuvenate itself. It helps to lower your blood pressure and actually results in less eating — and not just because when you are sleeping you can't eat!

Following is the breakdown of how much sleep your child should get to function properly:

- Age 1–3 years: 12–14 hours a day
- Age 3– 6 years: 11–12 hours a day
- Age 7–12 years: 10–11 hours a day
- Age 12–18 years: 8.25–9.5 hours a day

Makes sure your child gets enough rest so you do too!

A Positive Attitude Is Crucial

Children who maintain a positive attitude simply do better and live a happier life. Teach your child that when he has a positive attitude, he can accomplish whatever he wants to do.

Teach your child to substitute "I won't" for "I can't." The first suggests a choice while the second suggests inadequacy. Let your child know that alone or with help, he can do anything he wants.

Make it clear to your child that negative thinking is a choice as well. He can feel bad about a situation, or he can choose to get over it and remind himself that the situation is just temporary.

Helping a child learn a new skill also increases his self-confidence and self-worth and makes him feel more positive about himself and his world.

Finally, the best way to make your child feel really good about himself is to constantly remind him with words and hugs that he is loved.

One of my favorite sayings goes like this: "Someday we will laugh about this. Why not now?"

Appendix

Additional Resources

· ·

*Y*ou can find many online resources for more information. Here, I offer the best of them, grouped together as resources for prediabetes, resources for nutrition, and resources for exercise.

Resources for Prediabetes

The **American Diabetes Association** has all kinds of information on prediabetes, diabetes, nutrition, exercise, and so forth at www.diabetes.org. You will find some key articles on:

- Nutrition
- Fitness
- Lifestyle and prevention

Medline Plus has pages and pages of health topics in multiple languages that can be found at http://medlineplus.gov/. Just click on "Health Topics" and then "Metabolic Problems." There you will find articles on:

- Bariatric surgery
- Diabetes
- Diabetes complications
- Hypoglycemia
- Metabolic syndrome
- Obesity
- Obesity in children

Mayo Clinic has a lot of information on prediabetes, as well as diabetes. Go to `www.mayoclinic.com/health/prediabetes/DS00624/DSECTION=symptoms`. There you can find the following prediabetes information:

- Definition
- Symptoms
- Causes
- Risk factors
- When to seek medical advice
- Tests and diagnosis
- Treatment and drugs
- Prevention
- Alternative medicine

WebMD has a large amount of material on prediabetes at `http://diabetes.webmd.com/guide/prediabetes`. You can find:

- Overview and facts
- Symptoms and types
- Diagnosis and tests
- Treatment and care
- Living and management
- Support and resources

National Diabetes Education Program, a partnership of the National Institutes of Health, the Centers for Disease Control, and more than 200 public and private organizations, has information on all aspects of prediabetes and diabetes at `www.ndep.nih.gov/am-i-at-risk/index.aspx`. In particular you can click on these topics:

- Diabetes risk factors
- Diabetes is preventable
- Take small steps to prevent diabetes

You can also view these publications:

- "Small Steps, Big Rewards. Your GAME PLAN to Prevent Type 2 Diabetes: Information for Patients"
- "It's Not Too Late to Prevent Diabetes"
- "More than 50 Ways to Prevent Diabetes"

Resources for Nutrition

Recipes that are developed for people with diabetes are also helpful for people with prediabetes (or healthy people, for that matter).

Diabetic Cooking Magazine at www.diabeticcooking.com is filled with recipes for:

- ✔ Main dishes
- ✔ Desserts
- ✔ Food for kids
- ✔ Appetizers

You can also subscribe to the paper version of the magazine. Complete nutritional information is provided for every recipe.

Diabetic-recipes.com at www.diabetic-recipes.com has more than 800 diabetic and heart-healthy recipes. It also provides more than 200 menus for every occasion. You can search by the ingredient you want to use and come up with multiple choices. For example, if you choose "chicken" and "recipes," you are taken to a page of chicken recipes and can choose from:

- ✔ Apple and Thyme Chicken
- ✔ Apple, Rosemary and Thyme Chicken Baked in Parchment
- ✔ Asian Soup with Shredded Chicken and Rice
- ✔ Baked Chicken with Onions, Raisins and Sunflower Seeds
- ✔ And many, many others

Each recipe has complete nutritional information.

Cooksrecipes.com, found at www.cooksrecipes.com/category/diabetic. html, has more than 400 delicious recipes that emphasize low fat, low sugar, and high nutrition. The recipes include complete nutritional information.

Diabetic-lifestyle.com at www.diabetic-lifestyle.com also provides numerous recipes with nutritional information, as well as cooking tips, recipes just for kids, and recipes for entertaining. Complete nutritional information is included. The people who run this site also publish the *Cleveland Clinic Healthy Heart Lifestyle and Cookbook.*

Resources for Exercise

Diabetes Exercise and Sports Association at www.diabetes-exercise. org exists to enhance the quality of life for people with diabetes through exercise and physical fitness. Some of its features include:

- About Diabetes
- Be Active! Be Fit! Be Healthy!
- Ask the Athletes
- Ask the Experts
- Message Board

This association has an annual North American Conference in June and publishes *The Challenge Magazine* on a seasonal basis featuring articles about diabetes and sports.

Each one of the sites I describe in the "Resources for Prediabetes" section in this appendix also features discussions of diabetes and physical activity because physical activity is central to good health.

Index

• *E* •

• *Q* •

• *R* •

Business/Accounting & Bookkeeping

Bookkeeping For Dummies
978-0-7645-9848-7

eBay Business
All-in-One For Dummies,
2nd Edition
978-0-470-38536-4

Job Interviews
For Dummies,
3rd Edition
978-0-470-17748-8

Resumes For Dummies,
5th Edition
978-0-470-08037-5

Stock Investing
For Dummies,
3rd Edition
978-0-470-40114-9

Successful Time
Management
For Dummies
978-0-470-29034-7

Computer Hardware

BlackBerry For Dummies,
3rd Edition
978-0-470-45762-7

Computers For Seniors
For Dummies
978-0-470-24055-7

iPhone For Dummies,
2nd Edition
978-0-470-42342-4

Laptops For Dummies,
3rd Edition
978-0-470-27759-1

Macs For Dummies,
10th Edition
978-0-470-27817-8

Cooking & Entertaining

Cooking Basics
For Dummies,
3rd Edition
978-0-7645-7206-7

Wine For Dummies,
4th Edition
978-0-470-04579-4

Diet & Nutrition

Dieting For Dummies,
2nd Edition
978-0-7645-4149-0

Nutrition For Dummies,
4th Edition
978-0-471-79868-2

Weight Training
For Dummies,
3rd Edition
978-0-471-76845-6

Digital Photography

Digital Photography
For Dummies,
6th Edition
978-0-470-25074-7

Photoshop Elements 7
For Dummies
978-0-470-39700-8

Gardening

Gardening Basics
For Dummies
978-0-470-03749-2

Organic Gardening
For Dummies,
2nd Edition
978-0-470-43067-5

Green/Sustainable

Green Building
& Remodeling
For Dummies
978-0-470-17559-0

Green Cleaning
For Dummies
978-0-470-39106-8

Green IT For Dummies
978-0-470-38688-0

Health

Diabetes For Dummies,
3rd Edition
978-0-470-27086-8

Food Allergies
For Dummies
978-0-470-09584-3

Living Gluten-Free
For Dummies
978-0-471-77383-2

Hobbies/General

Chess For Dummies,
2nd Edition
978-0-7645-8404-6

Drawing For Dummies
978-0-7645-5476-6

Knitting For Dummies,
2nd Edition
978-0-470-28747-7

Organizing For Dummies
978-0-7645-5300-4

SuDoku For Dummies
978-0-470-01892-7

Home Improvement

Energy Efficient Homes
For Dummies
978-0-470-37602-7

Home Theater
For Dummies,
3rd Edition
978-0-470-41189-6

Living the Country Lifestyle
All-in-One For Dummies
978-0-470-43061-3

Solar Power Your Home
For Dummies
978-0-470-17569-9

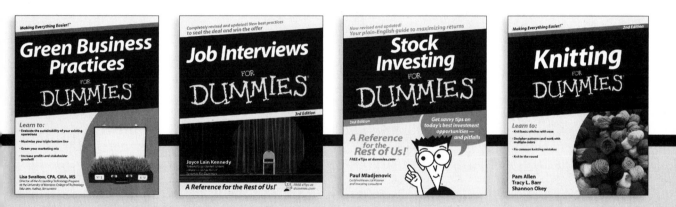

Internet

Blogging For Dummies,
2nd Edition
978-0-470-23017-6

eBay For Dummies,
6th Edition
978-0-470-49741-8

Facebook For Dummies
978-0-470-26273-3

Google Blogger
For Dummies
978-0-470-40742-4

Web Marketing
For Dummies,
2nd Edition
978-0-470-37181-7

WordPress For Dummies,
2nd Edition
978-0-470-40296-2

Language & Foreign Language

French For Dummies
978-0-7645-5193-2

Italian Phrases
For Dummies
978-0-7645-7203-6

Spanish For Dummies
978-0-7645-5194-9

Spanish For Dummies,
Audio Set
978-0-470-09585-0

Macintosh

Mac OS X Snow Leopard
For Dummies
978-0-470-43543-4

Math & Science

Algebra I For Dummies
978-0-7645-5325-7

Biology For Dummies
978-0-7645-5326-4

Calculus For Dummies
978-0-7645-2498-1

Chemistry For Dummies
978-0-7645-5430-8

Microsoft Office

Excel 2007 For Dummies
978-0-470-03737-9

Office 2007 All-in-One
Desk Reference
For Dummies
978-0-471-78279-7

Music

Guitar For Dummies,
2nd Edition
978-0-7645-9904-0

iPod & iTunes
For Dummies,
6th Edition
978-0-470-39062-7

Piano Exercises
For Dummies
978-0-470-38765-8

Parenting & Education

Parenting For Dummies,
2nd Edition
978-0-7645-5418-6

Type 1 Diabetes
For Dummies
978-0-470-17811-9

Pets

Cats For Dummies,
2nd Edition
978-0-7645-5275-5

Dog Training For Dummies,
2nd Edition
978-0-7645-8418-3

Puppies For Dummies,
2nd Edition
978-0-470-03717-1

Religion & Inspiration

The Bible For Dummies
978-0-7645-5296-0

Catholicism For Dummies
978-0-7645-5391-2

Women in the Bible
For Dummies
978-0-7645-8475-6

Self-Help & Relationship

Anger Management
For Dummies
978-0-470-03715-7

Overcoming Anxiety
For Dummies
978-0-7645-5447-6

Sports

Baseball For Dummies,
3rd Edition
978-0-7645-7537-2

Basketball For Dummies,
2nd Edition
978-0-7645-5248-9

Golf For Dummies,
3rd Edition
978-0-471-76871-5

Web Development

Web Design All-in-One
For Dummies
978-0-470-41796-6

Windows Vista

Windows Vista
For Dummies
978-0-471-75421-3

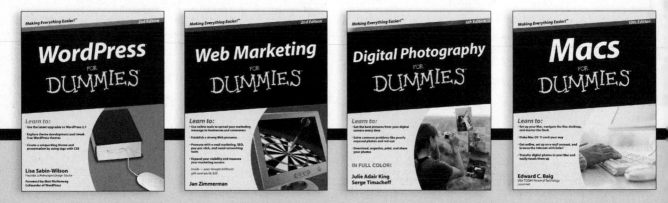

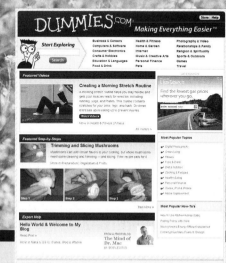
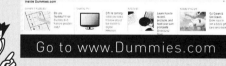

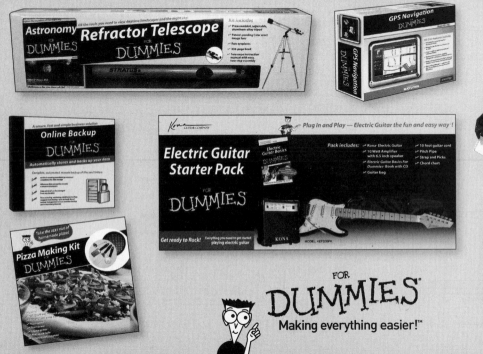
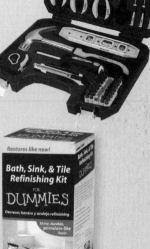